Blue Eyeshadow Should Absolutely Be Illegal

Third Edition—Revised and Updated

Other books by Paula Begoun to order from Beginning Press:

Don't Go to the Cosmetics Counters Without Me —
An Eye Opening Guide to Brand Name Cosmetics

To order, please send a check for $10.95, plus $1.50 for shipping and handling, to:

Beginning Press
5418 South Brandon
Seattle, Washington 98118

Blue Eyeshadow Should Absolutely Be Illegal

Third Edition—Revised and Updated

By Paula Begoun

Beginning Press

Editor: Sheree Bykofsky
Copy Editors: Susan M. Grossman and Judy Steer
Art Direction & Production: Lasergraphics
Cover Design: Patrick Howe
Photography: Bill Cannon
Makeup Artistry: Paula Begoun
Typography: Lasergraphics
Printed in the United States by Publishers Press, Salt Lake City, Utah

Copyright © 1985, 1988, 1992 by Paula Begoun
Beginning Press
5418 South Brandon
Seattle, Washington 98118

First Edition: January 1986
Second Edition: November 1988
Third Edition: February 1992
10 9 8 7 6 5 4 3 2 1
ISBN 1-877988-04-9

This book is distributed to the United States book trade by
Publishers Group West
4065 Hollis Street
Emeryville, CA 94608
(800) 788-3123

and to the Canadian book trade by
Raincoast Books Limited
112 East 3rd Avenue
Vancouver, B.C. V5T 1C8
CANADA
(604) 873-6581

Dedication

To consumer reporters everywhere who make
the world a safer place to shop.

Newsletter

If you are interested in receiving subscription information about Paula Begoun's *Cosmetic Update Newsletter*, available in June of 1992, just write to Beginning Press using the form on the next page, and we will send you the information as soon as it is available.

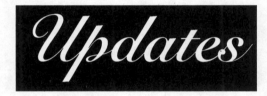

Beginning Press • 5418 South Brandon • Seattle, WA 98118

Publisher's Note

Chapter 1
What You Need to Know to Get Started

If every cosmetics company is promising the same thing—wrinkle-free, younger-looking skin—then either they're all telling the truth and except for the price it doesn't matter what products you buy, or they're all lying, and you shouldn't buy any of it.

Don't Go to the Cosmetics Counter Without This Book Either ...

It seems hard to believe that this is my third edition of *Blue Eyeshadow Should Be Illegal*. I wrote the first edition more than eight years ago. To say the least, a lot has happened over those eight years, both to the cosmetics industry and to me.

A major event for me was writing *Don't Go to the Cosmetics Counter Without Me—An Eye Opening Guide to Brand Name Cosmetics*. I reviewed more than 5,000 cosmetics from more than thirty major lines. The research was difficult because getting information from cosmetics counter personnel, as you have probably experienced yourself, is most definitely a struggle. After finishing the research for *Don't Go to the Cosmetics Counter Without Me*, I realized that several things had changed in my attitude and approach to skin care and makeup application. It seemed apparent that I would need to go back to the word processor once more and bring *Blue Eyeshadow Should Be Illegal* into the nineties.

Before we go any further, let me explain that *Don't Go to the Cosmetics Counter Without Me* is a brand name guide to buying specific cosmetic products. Like its predecessors, this edition of *Blue Eyeshadow Should Be Illegal* is a manual that will show you how to apply makeup and develop a reliable skin care routine of your own. In spite of the distinct differences between the books, each offers a revealing insight into the misleading information that is so rampant in the cosmetics industry. It is almost redundant and clichéd to suggest that cosmetics advertising, in both fashion magazines and television infomercials, and the cosmetics counters are not the places to find information about skin care or makeup application. But more about that later.

Among the events that made me decide to update *Blue Eyeshadow* were the personal and professional changes I had weathered over the eight years since I wrote the original version. Some of the transformations in my life were simply chronological: I'm fast approaching forty, my hair is graying, my face has wrinkles it didn't have before, and there is a certain sound I make when sitting down (or getting up) after a long day that I didn't make when I was younger. These physical changes and my feelings about them have had an impact on the way I work with my own makeup and skin care routines.

I wouldn't say the alterations in my attitudes and ideas about makeup application and skin care are necessarily radical; rather, they are more practical and realistic for a wider range of women than they used to be.

How could I not change? The life experiences swirling around my nearing forty have altered my feelings about the world of cosmetics—but I haven't responded to growing up the way the cosmetics companies would have me respond. They want me to feel insecure and despondent about the changes in my skin, hair, and appearance. The way the ads are designed, I am expected to look in the mirror, run my fingers anxiously over my skin, and lament the fact that I don't look like the eighteen-year-old models in the photographs. The more insecure I am, the more likely I am to spend a lot of money on products that offer the promise of youth and beauty. The products may not deliver on their vague, ambiguous claims and promises, but from the viewpoint of many women, buying some amount of hope (in the shape of a well-designed cosmetic product) is better than feeling hopeless for free. At least that's what the cosmetics industry is banking on.

Well, I feel neither depressed nor insecure about the way I look. I also don't believe that wasting money on products that advertise hope but can't deliver will make anyone feel better—at least, not women who know better. And we are all beginning or wanting to know better, or else you wouldn't have picked up this book and read this far.

> The products may not deliver on their vague, ambiguous claims and promises, but from the viewpoint of many women, buying some amount of hope is better than feeling hopeless for free.

There is also one other factor that affected my decision to revise *Blue Eyeshadow*. Over the years I have received thousands of letters from women who have read my books, and I have a much better understanding now of what many women want from their cosmetics, why they get confused at the cosmetics counter, and, most important, what makes them look and feel good and what doesn't. This new *Blue Eyeshadow Should Be Illegal* will attempt to straighten all that out and incorporate the new things I've learned along the way. The makeup application part of this book will teach you what colors look best on what skin tones, why you should use different products for different skin types, what makeup designs look best with your particular life-style, and how to apply your makeup quickly and beautifully. The skin care section discusses how to best take care of your skin, what skin care ingredients work with specific skin types, and how to decide what to do when problems arise. In both the makeup and skin care section I will take great care in letting you know the differences between what the cosmetics industry wants you to believe and what is perhaps a more rational and realistic way to think about your skin and appearance.

One more point about change. Of all the things that I've noticed have changed over the years, the area in which the least change has taken place is the cosmetics industry. Actually, that isn't 100 percent true. The cosmetics industry loves me even less than they did eight years ago. (I often wonder if this is what Ralph Nader has gone through with insurance companies and the automobile industry.) Writing my last book, *Don't Go to the Cosmetics Counter Without Me*, definitely didn't help my relationship with the cosmetics industry.

One of my favorite letters came from a group of saleswomen who sold Borghese products. They wanted me to know that all my positive comments about Borghese were truthful and wonderful but that the negative comments were totally inaccurate and irresponsible. It was amazing to me that they thought I could be right about anything when it came to their products. When I asked them to review my specific complaints about their ingredients and claims, they didn't respond. I also received a long letter from The Body Shop (a chain of "natural" cosmetics stores) wherein it was stated that many of my assertions about the shop's products were likewise incorrect. When I asked to see the company's research documentation, however, so that I could reconsider my position (I'm always willing to reconsider my position), the company did not respond.

The letters that have meant the most to me did not come from the cosmetics industry. I've received so many letters from consumers who say I've saved them from wasting money at the cosmetics counters and saved their skin to boot. If I can do the same for you, all of this will have been worthwhile. And as long as the cosmetics industry continues doing what they do, then it is important that I continue doing what I do.

If you already have a good sense of what kinds of products you want to use, then *Don't Go to the Cosmetics Counter Without Me* will tell you the specific products that work best. If you want more information about what skin care routines work best for your skin type, what colors look best for your skin coloring, and detailed information about how and why particular cosmetic products work, then this edition of *Blue Eyeshadow Should Be Illegal* will tell you exactly what you need to know.

Why Do I Have a Thing About Blue Eyeshadow?

For the most part it's an aesthetic call, but I'm also taking a stand against the misleading information that abounds at the cosmetics counters. Blue eyeshadow—specifically, bright, opaque, or iridescent blue eyeshadow—and I haven't had a good relationship since the late 1960s. This issue has nothing to do with allergic reactions or health; it remains an issue of fashion and misinformation at the cosmetics counters. Women are nudged into purchasing many products that are just plain wrong for them. Sometimes the women themselves are mistaken about what looks best on them, but other times they are misled by poorly informed salespeople.

No woman should be sold bright blue or green eyeshadow. She should also never be sold pink, orange, or green foundation; pink, orange, or green highlighter; white or orange powder; iridescent eyeshadows; or greasy eye pencils. You never (or rarely) see these things on models in fashion magazines, and you would be hard put to find a professional makeup artist who disagrees with me. Would any fashion designer of any kind ever put a model in glaring eyeshadow, smeary eye pencil, or heavy, unnatural foundation?

Suffice it to say, and I will try not to say it again, blue eyeshadow represents what is still going awry at the cosmetics counter. All too often we buy cosmetics that do not enhance our own beauty. What I will do throughout these following chapters is explain how to avoid making those mistakes so you never have to be a glamour "don't" again or, worse, waste your money at the cosmetics counters.

Fashion Magazine Mania

Once we accept the fact that most fashion magazines do not offer the most objective information about skin care and makeup, we can begin to use them for what they do best. Fashion magazines are a remarkably reliable source for learning what is fashionable and what isn't. Yet so frequently, regardless of how many of these magazines we read per year, we still purchase many colors and products that completely negate what the magazines show us is attractive.

Many of you know by now that I have strong feelings about the content of most fashion magazines. Separate from the ads, the editorial sections and the stories about cosmetics are frequently not what I would call impartial. You've seen the banners on the covers for such enticing, potentially compelling stories as "The Truth About Wrinkle Creams", "The Most Common Myths About Skin", or "The Skin Care Experts Tell You What Is Best For You." Doesn't it sound as if you are about to find out some shocking truths about skin care products?

In reality, many of these articles are not revealing, and they offer no insights that differ from the cosmetics industry's point of view. What I have found is that most of these editorials blatantly support or endorse every product the cosmetics companies make. These articles are written in such a way that the information doesn't offend advertisers. The expert quoted often works for a particular cosmetics company—hardly what I would call an objective authority! Personally, I know what has happened to some of the interviews I've done with magazines: my "controversial" facts either get edited out or are eliminated altogether.

As a rule of thumb, when you're reading any story in a fashion magazine that is about the beauty business and an expert from a cosmetics or pharmaceutical company is quoted, take the information with a very, very large grain of salt. Cosmetics company representatives or pharmaceutical representatives are not in the business of offering inside information that would keep you from buying one of their products. For the most part, you can be fairly certain that it is not in the fashion magazine's best interest to be relating entirely objective information about the cosmetics industry.

Skin care is one of the major areas where magazines find themselves financially at odds with the truth about what cosmetics can and can't do. Cosmetics companies spend a lot of money taking out pages and pages of very expensive ads. If a cosmetics company claims or implies in a $60,000 ad that a certain product can eliminate your wrinkles, the editors would be downright foolish to include articles telling you that wrinkle creams don't work. That would not be good business. As the advertiser of that wrinkle cream, you would only have to threaten to take your business someplace else. That is exactly what can happen. That is why many of the articles seem to support what the cosmetics industry wants you to know and what they want you to think.

I should mention that many fashion magazines do offer beauty tips that do not directly endorse or negate cosmetics companies' claims. These tips, even when I don't agree with them (such as making your own facial masks or placing tea bags and cucumbers over the eyes to reduce puffiness), can save you money. Just recently I read an article in *Allure* magazine that I thought was remarkably objective and insightful. They stated boldly that cellulite creams and placenta extracts were cosmetic gimmicks. Thank you, *Allure* magazine, my subscription check is in the mail.

On television and in magazines, just be aware that advertising dollars often control the information you are getting. When advertisers control the editorial content of the programming, there isn't much you or I can do about it—except be more knowledgeable.

Note: *In all fairness to fashion magazines, I want to state that the articles they publish are often engrossing, well written, and exceptionally helpful. There are many money-saving, convenient, and challenging ideas presented. I learn a lot from these journals and enjoy reading them. Of course, I generally wince at much of the cosmetics information, but that is understandable.*

Ads Make Pretty Pictures and That's About It

If American consumers would come to terms with what advertising is truly all about, we would all make much better decisions about what we buy. In other words, you can't believe everything (or, as some consumer reporters might warn, anything) an ad says about the product advertised. Nowhere is this more relevant than in the cosmetics industry. The statements and slogans you read in ads or on the packaging do not tell you what you need to know in order to make a decision about buying a particular product. Phrases like "Dermatologist Tested" or "Laboratory Tested" do not tell you who the dermatologist was or who was in the lab doing the research. It also doesn't provide you with the results of the study. What if a cosmetics company tested its own products on only two people, its president and vice-president, and then asserted it got positive results? Can you really base a decision on that data, more or less extrapolate what will be true for you as one of the millions of women who may buy the product? You can't, but most of the time the companies would have you misinterpret such flimsy or meaningless claims.

The latest outrageous cosmetics industry advertising ploy comes in the form of television ads that show a before and after close-up of a woman's skin after a product is applied to "prove" that the woman's wrinkles have retreated permanently. These ads make me want to call the Food and Drug Administration, which regulates the industry, and ask them to tune in. The best word to describe such an ad is *absurd*. The one I saw the other day was so obviously contrived that I wondered who would believe it? The before and after pictures were shot in different lighting. Guess which lighting was more flattering? In the before picture, the woman's eyes were slightly closed. In the after close-up, her eyes were wide open. Judging from the vast number of ads that are showing up on every cable station, I can only conclude unhappily that people must be buying this nonsense along with the products. To further bolster consumer confidence, the ads depict interviews with women who are thrilled with the product. Remember that these are advertorials—paid advertisements—and these women are not there to be objective, but are probably being paid for their time.

At the cosmetics counters there are often impressively designed, scientific-looking brochures showing how well a product works on the skin. You might see, for example, a microscopic close-up of a patch of skin with an explanation of how bad it looks. Beside it is a close-up patch of the same skin after the cream is applied. See how wonderfully the product worked? The deception here is that you are not given enough "before" information. For example, how dry was the skin before the product was applied? Did the woman have severely dry skin? Had she not used a moisturizer for several days or several weeks before the test was done? Had she just used some irritating soaps or astringents just before the picture was taken to make sure the skin looked really dry and flaky? In that case, any moisturizing cream would make the skin look much improved. Just because information looks scientific doesn't mean it is.

Be aware of the vast difference between the information advertising provides and what one might call objective information. Advertising is one-sided. There are no negatives in ads, unless they are about the competition's products. The truth about almost all products on the market, whether from the cosmetics industry or some other industry, is that they all have their pros and cons. The job for every consumer is not to be swayed by advertising alone. Be realistic. It is not the task of the company paying for the ad or of the salesperson selling you the product to do anything but portray the product in absolutely glowing, positive terms. It is, however, the consumer's job to search out as much impartial information from independent sources as possible. You might still buy the product advertised, but at least you would have some real facts to base your decision on and not just pretty pictures and creatively written words.

> If every product actually contained the secret or magical combination of ingredients that was going to cure or eliminate wrinkles or other skin problems, then it wouldn't matter what product you bought.

As far as cosmetics are concerned, the only candid information to be found is on the ingredients label. It won't surprise you when I tell you that the only part of the cosmetic product that never gets its picture in the magazine or air time on television is the ingredients label. I know ingredients labels can be difficult to understand, but this is one of the only areas that can get you safely through a cosmetics counter encounter. I'll give you more specifics about ingredients labels later.

Whether or not you ever start paying attention to ingredients, it would help you immensely if you always remember the consumer reporter's creed: if it sounds too good to be true, it is. The other axiom to adopt is that there are no miracles out there. Keep this thought in mind the next time you are approached with the "latest" cosmetic wonder product: if every product actually contained the secret or magical combination of ingredients that was going to cure or eliminate wrinkles or other skin problems, then it wouldn't matter what product you bought. You might tell yourself that the more expensive the product, the greater the possibility of finding the fountain of youth or a close facsimile. That would be nice—what's a few extra dollars if it means finding heaven in a bottle?—except that almost all of us have bought expensive products at one time or another that haven't worked. There are things that can be done to make sure you take very good care of your skin, but that has little to do with the exaggerated, absurd claims of most cosmetics companies. Even if you can afford the price tag for some products, wasting money is never desirable.

One more point about cosmetic ads: beautiful models are beautiful not because they know anything about skin care or makeup, but because they happen to be beautiful! I'd like to share with you a letter I received that I believe reflects what many women identify with when they see a stunning model in a cosmetics ad or in a fashion layout.

Dear Paula,

I have some ideas you may want to use for your next book. Are you familiar with fashion magazines that say on the cover, "Beauty Secrets of Top Models?" I'd love to read a book that had beautiful women that told exactly what they use on their skin, such as foundations and moisturizers. These women have great skin and a good makeup system. Christie Brinkley is the spokesmodel for Cover Girl makeup. Who better than her would know the best of their line?

Vicky
Burbank, CA

My response was as follows:

Dear Vicky,

You seem to have a belief that famous people or beautiful models know something about makeup or have found products they like a lot, and that is why they look good. Neither of those points is necessarily true. First, celebrities look good because they look good. That's why they have gotten somewhere in our media-saturated world. A pretty face (particularly for a woman) is one of the major reasons they are successful as an actress or model, not because they know anything about cosmetics. Good skin is one of the assets (besides a good figure) that is required for success. Famous people are not necessarily any happier with their makeup or skin care products than you are; they can simply afford to waste more money in their search. And, bottom line, when celebrities have their pictures taken, makeup artists and top-notch photographers are always involved. When I worked as a makeup artist years ago and did many personalities' faces, I can promise you that the way many of them did their makeup was more often than not terrible. That's why makeup artists are always backstage or present at a photo shoot. The problem with your other point is that a spokesperson for a particular cosmetics line, hair care line, or type of gasoline, for that matter, is not necessarily an expert about those products. What that celebrity knows is how to have her agent work out the best deal. Lending your face to represent a company has more to do with a three-million-dollar contract than it has to do with use or belief in a product line.

I remember when I was first trying to get my original makeup book published I was told by several publishers that because I wasn't Linda Evans or Brooke Shields, women wouldn't want to read what I have to say. After selling more than 250,000 books I know that this attitude is changing more and more. Women know, or are learning, that actresses know about acting and models know about modeling and not necessarily anything about the products they're advertising.

My advice to Vicky and to everyone is to rethink your attitude about cosmetics advertising (or advertising in general), and you may start being less swayed by slick ads and pretty faces and more by practical consumer decisions.

Reading Between the Lines

One of the questions I am asked most frequently is what about truth in advertising? How can the cosmetics companies get away with what they say? The Food and Drug Administration (FDA) does, to some extent, control false advertising or the false claims on the packaging, but that is easy enough for the cosmetics industry to circumvent. Except for the ingredients label, which is carefully regulated by the FDA, all other parts of the packaging and advertising are subject to advertising strategy and clever, evasive wording. The job for the cosmetics, advertising, and marketing departments is to make a product sound like it can do what the FDA says a cosmetic can't do (because if the cosmetic could do what the ad implied it would be classified as a drug and be regulated much more stringently). Cosmetics companies can't legally use phrases that directly state or promise that a permanent change to the skin will take place when a product is used. But there are plenty of ways to make something sound permanent to the consumer without sounding permanent to the Food and Drug Administration.

In essence, whenever you read an ad or a label on a cosmetic product, there are three very different messages being sent at the same time. First, there is the message the cosmetics company wants you (the consumer) to get about the product. Second, there is the message that the cosmetics company needs the Food and Drug Administration to approve. Third, there is the truth about the product. Too often these three conflicting messages are eons apart.

My favorite example these days is cellulite cream, one of the most bogus cosmetics to be sold to date. Composed primarily of normal skin care ingredients, these creams supposedly remove cellulite when you rub or pound the stuff into your thighs. The saleswoman who sold me the Lancôme product I bought carried on and on about what a difference it had made to her thighs. The language on the container reads like this:

Cellulite "Relief" Gel

A state-of-the-art transport system in a featherweight gel that delivers special hydrators, cellulite specifics, and a modern mix of natural botanicals where skin surface areas need help most: thighs, hips, upper arms, derriere. Provides time-released ingredients for up to 24 hours after application. So you only have to use it once a day.

Notice that the word *relief* is in quotes. Once a word is quoted, no strict dictionary definition can be applied. No definition means you (the consumer) can think anything you want about what is implied about relieving your cellulite with this product. "Relief" to the consumer probably means "gets rid of" or "reduces the number of bumps on" the thighs. When the Food and Drug Administration says to the company that made the product, What do you mean by "relief"? the executives can say that they meant the consumer would feel better about her cellulite after using the product. No, it doesn't get rid of cellulite, but a woman might feel "relieved" after using it. Why not? Skin feels good after creams are massaged into it and people feel relieved when they take action to alleviate a problem. Now that is radically different from what *you* thought was meant by the phrase "cellulite 'relief'."

Farther down the label, as we analyze the rest of what I call cosmetic mystery language, the term "cellulite specifics" is a total mystery to me, as it should be, because there is no such thing. If you wanted to know what the term meant, you'd have to ask Lancôme—or you could guess. *Botanicals* is another word for plants, but why *modern*? I suppose these plants were picked recently as opposed to a thousand years ago. *Featherweight* is very subjective; all gels and creams can be called featherweight. *Time-released* ingredients and the *state-of-the-art transport system* refer to liposomes. Liposomes are a good moisturizing ingredient, and they are indeed time-released, which helps moisturize the skin for a longer period of time than normal, but that won't change cellulite one iota.

What does this cellulite gel really do? According to the ingredients, it contains some moisturizers, a peeling agent, and oils. Will any of that burn fat from the outside in? Of course not. If it could, none of us would have visible fat anywhere. In fact, we would rub it on all parts of our body that bulged where we didn't want it to bulge, and the bulge would slowly disappear. We'd use it instead of dieting. But then again, this product claim never used the word *fat* anywhere; it is alluded to, but that is all. According to the cosmetics industry cellulite exists and fat is different from cellulite. According to the medical community and everyone not associated with products designed to get rid of cellulite, the dimples on your thighs and buttocks indicate excess fat, plain and simple.

Let's examine another label just for the sake of doing this helpful exercise one more time. My personal favorite group of products that promise the world and deliver little are wrinkle creams. The ads for Time Zone™ products by Estée Lauder are a perfect example:

Time Zone
Moisture Recharging Complex

It's a rich, airy creme that provides an immediate hydrating boost and helps skin retain moisture longer. It protects against damaging UV rays. This helps your skin resist forming lines and wrinkles for years longer than you'd expect.

Time Zone Eyes
Ultra-hydrating Complex

Just for your ultra-delicate eye area, here's a liqui-creme with the same unique technology that also calms fine lines. Makes dark circles and puffiness seem to disappear. We'll even show you the data if you like.

The claims in these ads are subtler than those for the cellulite cream. Time Zone sounds good, but there is nothing special about it. The name implies that it prevents the skin from growing up. Companies have more latitude in naming their products than in making false claims about them. Don't be seduced by creative names. The term *rich* means *creamy*, which this product is but not more so than others I've tested. *Airy* means *lightweight*, but likewise it's not lighter than other similar products. The line about an immediate hydrating boost means the product contains water and oil (water is what hydration refers to), which is the exact same claim that can be made by any other moisturizer. A moisturizer helps the skin retain water—plain and simple.

The comment about protecting the skin from the sun is overblown, but that is a very popular thing for skin care products to do these days. If there is a drop of sunscreen in the product, usually Sun Protecting Factor (SPF) of 8 or less, the claim is made that it can protect the face from the harmful effects of the sun. And yet I have not interviewed a dermatologist who doesn't say that in order for a sunscreen to be effective against the sun, you must use an SPF of 15 or greater, and you must reapply the sunscreen frequently. Time Zone does not have an SPF of 15, and because you will probably wear it under your makeup, you won't be reapplying it. To suggest that Time Zone does anything to change or improve the way the skin will age in regard to the sun or otherwise is not accurate.

Having said all that, I still think Time Zone can work as a good moisturizer. I think it's overpriced, but that has nothing to do with whether or not it is a good product. The overblown claims and vague wording get in the way of what really makes this product good: moisturizing ingredients such as oils, hyaluronic acid, cholesterol esters, and polysaccharides. But if the ads for these products were to concentrate on just ingredients, they wouldn't sound anywhere near as interesting or be that different from a hundred other moisturizers. And that's because they're not. It would be more truthful but definitely not as interesting.

Actually, I can go on and on with these examples—there are literally thousands of them—but rather than going product by product, which is what I do in *Don't Go to the Cosmetics Counter Without Me*, I'm going to analyze some standard cosmetic phrases and expressions. Some of my favorites, designed to sweep the consumer into a buying stupor, follow.

"Anti-aging"

The only products that get to make this claim are those that contain a sunscreen. The sun causes skin to wrinkle. Sunscreen blocks the effect of the sun on the skin and therefore slows the skin's aging process. Besides sunscreen, there is nothing in the world of cosmetic creams and lotions that has any anti-aging potential. When it comes to preventing wrinkles, not all sunscreens are equally effective. As I said before, most dermatologists would argue that, unless a product contains a sunscreen of SPF 15 or greater, it isn't worth much for protecting the skin from the sun. If a product contains any amount of sunscreen, however, it is permitted by law to make this misleading claim.

"Closest to your skin's own strengthening lipids"

Lipids are fats, nothing more, and skin contains lipids (the sebum your skin secretes as oil is a lipid). The term *strengthen* can mean that the lipids augment, or add to, your own lipids. Any fat added to the skin will do that, and that is good for dry skin. If you read *strengthen* to mean that it will tone up or support your skin, then you've read it wrong.

"Soothing botanicals"

Botanicals are simply plants, such as herbs and flowers, or extracts from the same in the form of oils or juices. In fact, *botanicals* is the nineties version of the well-used term *natural*. Is any of that soothing? For some skins I guess it can be, but the same can be said of cool water on the face; soothing isn't unique to botanicals. The claim is subjective, and by the way, you can be allergic to some botanicals.

"Soon expression lines appear smoother."

The operative word here is *appear*. What you think *appear smoother* means is one thing; what it means literally is something else. What "seems" or "appears" to be smoother to you may be different from what the cosmetics company really meant or from what someone else thinks. Besides, that claim can be attributed to any and all moisturizers. Dry skin can look more "superficially wrinkled"; put a moisturizer on, and dry skin can look smoother. That won't get rid of wrinkles, but then, that isn't what the ad said, it's just what it implied. Realize that if the lines actually were made smoother, surely they wouldn't settle for telling you that they just *appear* smoother.

"Superficial lines"

Watch out for the word *superficial*; it is a powerful cosmetic advertising tool. When you see the words *superficial* lines you can replace them with the words *temporary* lines or *those lines caused only by dryness*. Most products could make elaborate claims about superficial wrinkles and they would not be lying to you. Superficial wrinkles are those wrinkles caused by dryness. Superficial wrinkles go away when you put any moisturizer on, and that is wonderful. But, I repeat, but, superficial wrinkles are not the ones you are really worried about. Permanent wrinkles, like laugh lines, furrows between the eyes and on the forehead, and expression lines, are not eliminated by the use of any moisturizer. The word *superficial* is misleading because we want it to refer to the lines and wrinkles we are most concerned about and it doesn't.

"Start today and see a young tomorrow."

First, this line doesn't say that young has anything to do with you; rather it has to do with a tomorrow being young. So exactly what is a young tomorrow? Is the implication that tomorrow you will see a younger you? That's not what is said, but that's the impression you're supposed to get. Even if the phrase did say you would "see a younger you," how much younger are you supposed to see yourself tomorrow? Five minutes? An hour? A day? "See a young tomorrow" suggests something will happen to your wrinkles, but that is not *actually* what is being said; it's only what you *hope* is being said.

"Protects against damaging UV rays"

The product contains sunscreen. Period. And again, unless a product contains a sunscreen of SPF 15 or greater, the claim is useless and misleading. If the product doesn't state how much sunscreen it contains, then it is probably below an SPF of 8 or 6. That isn't enough to really protect you from the damaging rays of the sun.

"Just for your ultra-delicate eye area"

The advertiser may want you to use the eye cream only around your eyes so that you then have to buy a face lotion separately, but the ingredients of these products are rarely different enough to warrant the extra expense. Oftentimes the ingredients in the eye cream are actually heavier and greasier than those in the face lotion, although the salesperson will insist that the eye cream is formulated to be lighter than the face lotion. Test it out for yourself. When the face lotion feels and looks lighter than the eye cream, the ingredients will confirm that it is. The same cream would be usable for both face and eye areas. (The only time a special eye cream would be necessary is when the skin around the eyes is drier than the rest of the face.)

"Calms fine lines"

I never knew wrinkles needed calming. Were they overexcited in the first place? Is the suggestion that if your skin is stressed out it must look more wrinkly? There is no proof that stress affects the way the skin ages.

Anyway, if stress does affect wrinkles, I want to know how creams can reduce stress from the outside in.

"Makes dark circles and puffiness seem to disappear"
There's that word *seem*—watch out for it. There are no creams that can eliminate puffiness or dark circles. However, dry skin can *seem* puffier and darker. Any moisturizer applied over an eye area that is dehydrated will "seem" to be less dark and less puffy.

"Enriched with the sea's essential proteins"
Proteins from the sea? Is that like dead fish or something? Maybe they mean the proteins extracted from sea plants? Whatever it is, it can't affect the proteins in your skin.

"Dimpling seems to virtually disappear."
You'll start noticing the word *seem* more and more in cosmetics advertising once you start realizing that including this word (or the word *appear*) works as a disclaimer, negating the entire statement. The word sounds like a sweeping term, but it is there more for effect than for meaning. The word "virtually" is also a disclaimer. According to the dictionary *virtually* means "in effect, but not factually." So there is absolutely no guarantee from this statement that anything will change.

"Fresh, living seaweeds, which are rapidly frozen to retain their sea-born benefits"
This one sounds really good, doesn't it? It gives you the impression that if you open the container you will hear the ocean surf in the distance. Seaweed that is frozen is no longer alive, so what difference does it make if it was fresh in the first place? Once the seaweed is placed in the product, cooked and bottled and distributed all over the world for sale, do you think there is anything resembling seaweed left in the product? Let's say there are some seaweed nutrients left in the bottle. Is seaweed supposed to be some kind of miracle for the skin? If it is, why don't we just buy fresh seaweed and put that on our face? I include this one with all those statements that sound like you can put food or plants on the face and feed the skin. You can't. And the ads don't say that you can —they just imply it.

"Processed, packaged, and sealed under pharmaceutical conditions"
All cosmetics are made in this manner. This is not a special or unique service. Were you under the impression that other cosmetics were assembled in the middle of a junkyard?

"Deeply purified, visibly toned, and softened"

This describes how your face is supposed to feel after applying the product. When it comes to cleaning the face, you are supposed to believe that the skin is in need of a "deep" cleaning—that most skin problems are somehow related to dirty skin. If you just get it clean enough, then your problems will go away. That is not true. Besides, the ingredients that supposedly "deeply purify" the skin more times than not deeply dehydrate the skin. I asked many women and cosmeticians to comment, and *visibly toned* is a term that I could not get a consensus on. *Toned* to some women meant closed pores. No product can close pores. Most products that say they can tone the skin contain irritants that swell the skin and make it look closed for a few minutes. In another few minutes it's back to the way it was. There were others who felt *toned* skin meant something about better skin texture. In that regard, any product that contains emollients can make dry skin appear to have a smoother texture —dehydrated skin can look less smooth than normal or oily skin does. But the bottom line is that *toned* is an entirely subjective word that really tells you nothing, and it is used on all sorts of products with all sorts of ingredients for all sorts of skin types.

"Nighttime repair"

The suggestion here is that somehow this cream can help increase cell production. At night the skin automatically produces more skin cells than it does during the day. When claims about a cosmetic product being able to create new skin cells are made, the effect is microscopically insignificant. There is no convincing evidence that these creams make any difference in the appearance of the skin, given what naturally takes place at night in the skin. This is another one of those scientific-sounding claims that only work to attract naive consumers.

"Works like the fluids in your skin"

If you need some extra water in your skin because your skin is dry, putting a little moisturizer on it that contains water and oils will work like the water and oil fluids in your skin.

"Nourishing hydrobeads release vitamins and minerals."

You can't feed the skin from the outside in, and there is no evidence that vitamins and minerals can do anything for the surface of the skin. The word *hydrobeads* sounds like a special delivery system that can somehow transport these vitamins and minerals into the skin. They can't. Literally, *hydrobeads* means "beads of water." Big deal. There are a lot of these "microbeads" running around in cosmetics nowadays. It's a nineties gimmick, not a nineties scientific breakthrough for the skin.

"All at once the past is forgiven, the present improved, the future perfect."

This doesn't refer to anything specific, but it is wonderfully seductive. If it were a pill, we would eat it all day long. Sometimes ads don't really say anything about what the product does; they just imply that the product will do something, anything, that may be good for the skin.

"Microtargeted skin gel—rebuilding the skin's appearance"

Microtargeted is a good word. It sounds like this gel will zap just the area where you need it to work. If you have a wrinkle right next to your eye, no other area will be affected by the gel, right? That is what it sounds like, but that isn't what it really can do. It doesn't say that it can either; it leaves it to you to jump to that wrong conclusion. The term can be applied to anything. Microtarget just means "little center" or "little goal." What that has to do with the skin gel is anyone's guess.

"Test results reveal the cream beneficially affected the appearance of the skin surface."

Whose test results? In almost every case the cosmetics company is quoting their own results. Note that this is another subjective *appearance*, too—not what you would call a neutral source of information.

"In order for the products to achieve dramatic results you must use all of them; the skin must be properly conditioned to accept all the products in the line in order for any of the products to work."

This is one of my favorites because its purpose is to convince you to buy all the products. It is a classic sales technique. In essence what you are being told is that the wrinkle cream won't work unless all the other products are used first, so don't bother buying the wrinkle cream unless you are going to buy everything. In my years of reviewing skin care routines, I have never seen a cosmetic line with ingredients so unique that you couldn't substitute a dozen other products. But then again, cosmetics companies never want to talk about ingredients; they only want to talk in vague generalities. Moreover, the term to note here is *dramatic results*. What the cosmetics company considers *dramatic results* may be dramatically different from what you would really like to see the products do — even if you do buy and wear all of them.

"Dramatically diminishes wrinkles by penetrating the top layer of skin to create a balloon effect, pushing the skin out from beneath the surface."

I had a rough time deciphering this one. But after reading the ingredients, it was obvious that all the product could do was to irritate the skin, which would make it swell. Swollen skin can look temporarily less wrinkled. Of course, this ad didn't mention that most dermatologists warn against using products that irritate the skin on wrinkles, because the irritation can eventually make wrinkles worse. Ironic, isn't it, that many of the very products advertised as diminishing wrinkles can possibly make wrinkles more pronounced?

"The skin around the eye is thinner, with fewer oil glands, so it requires more hydration—this product will make the skin feel more resilient and make puffiness and bags subside."

It is true that the skin around the eye is thinner and has fewer oil glands and can be drier than the skin on the rest of the face, but that doesn't mean it needs more hydration; it needs more oil to keep the hydration (water) in. Any moisturizer can make this claim, because skin that is moist will feel more resilient and look less puffy.

"Realistic help is here."

Well, if ever a sentence said nothing, this is it. It's not at all clear what is meant by *realistic*. *Realistic* could mean "no help at all." The same applies to the word *help*. What I think is help and what they mean by help can be two entirely different things.

"Works with the microcirculation of your skin"

Works with is always a good phrase, but exactly what kind of work is it referring to? Microcirculation sounds very impressive. Yet all creams can technically affect the microcirculation of the skin. If the idea is to stimulate circulation, then any cream rubbed onto the skin can do that. It isn't the cream doing the stimulation, but your fingers rubbing the cream into your skin. Suggesting in an ad that—product or no product—all you need to do is massage your skin wouldn't sell very many products, so they say it this way. Sounds like macrocircumlocution to me (big double talk).

"Penetrates deeply into the layers of the skin"

Penetrates is one of the most misleading terms the cosmetic industry uses. Anything, if it is a small enough molecule, will penetrate the skin. Most moisturizers have too large a molecular structure to penetrate entirely into the skin. When a moisturizer can penetrate the skin, the word *layers* is frequently added to confound you. One layer of skin is so microscopically small, it is negligible. The cream can penetrate thousands of layers and still not have traveled anywhere. And even if the cream could penetrate deep into the skin, it would be partially absorbed and partially flushed out, which is what you would want it to do. You wouldn't want the skin to try and use the preservatives, fragrance, and coloring agents as well as the so-called beneficial ingredients. The entire concept assumes you can change the skin from the outside in by absorbing some benefit from the cream, and that is not possible from a cosmetic. If it were possible, the cosmetic would no longer be a cosmetic, it would be a drug, and as such would be subject to different FDA regulations.

"The skin's ability for self-rejuvenation is helped."

I'm not quite sure what they mean by self-rejuvenation. Rejuvenate means to restore youth. It sounds to me as if they want to imply you can make yourself look younger (and healthier). The same question applies here as before—how much youth is restored? A few minutes? A few hours? One week? Then again, it's suggested that it's the skin's natural ability to heal itself that is being aided. Cosmetics, by definition, don't heal.

"All natural" (or "all pure")

More than any other claim, this is the one consumers seem to love the most, which is probably why the cosmetics industry keeps it around. I wish I had a dime for every time a woman said to me, "Oh, yes, their product is 'all natural,' they use only 'pure' ingredients." *Natural* is still one of those great marketing terms that automatically sounds like what you're buying must be good for you. *Natural* conjures up images of health and safety—safe to use and healthy for the skin. Vitamins, herbs, and anything else that doesn't sound like a chemical qualifies as natural in this imaginary world—imaginary because *natural* has nothing intrinsically to do with health or herbs or good skin care.

Remember, too, that *natural* is not synonymous with *good*, *healthy*, or *safe*. I can think of many things that are natural that are anything but healthy or safe for the skin: ammonia, sulphuric acid, urine, formalde-hyde, glass, rock, and so on. Besides, many products made by companies boasting that their products are "all natural" contain preservatives and other synthetic ingredients that are about as far from natural (as we imagine it to mean) as you can get. These "unnatural" ingredients aren't necessarily bad for your skin; it's just that there is a difference between what you're really buying and what you thought you were buying. If buying a "natural" product made you feel that you were getting something that didn't contain all those nasty chemicals, think again. Whether or not a product is labeled "natural" does not tell you a thing about what you are buying. There are no specific guidelines surrounding what can or cannot be inside a "natural" product. Cosmetics called "natural" still contain preservatives, coloring agents, and all the other things you can think of that sound very unnatural.

"Hypoallergenic"

Hypoallergenic is one of my favorite cosmetic nonsense words. According to the dictionary, hypoallergenic means "less likely to cause an allergic reaction than other comparable products." There are several problems with this word and definition that make it a totally irrelevant concept. First, there are no guidelines to regulate what can and cannot be used in a so-called hypoallergenic product. Second, in 1978 the United States District Court of Appeals disallowed the term hypoallergenic as having any legal meaning. Third, who's to say what a comparable product is? And finally, there is no way a product, regardless of what it is called, can know what you, as an individual, will be allergic to. What makes me scratch and sneeze may be different from what makes you react similarly. Or where I scratch and sneeze, you may blotch and turn red. There is no way a hypoallergenic product can be universally less allergenic than another product. Knowing what will cause you to react is a hit-and-miss process of discovering what ingredients are problematic for you and you alone.

"Complexions looked smoother, felt better faster; their skin tone became more uniform and fine lines less noticeable."

This is supposedly a quote from a medical expert about a particular new cream. There are three basic problems with this statement: 1) Complexions looked smoother than what—than that of the person next to them—than they did ten seconds ago? Smoother is a vague, extremely subjective term. 2) Felt better faster than what? Than after using a different product, after using nothing, or after using something irritating on the skin? 3) Skin tone becoming more uniform and fine lines being less noticeable can be said about any moisturizer. Comparative terms used to compare something to nothing in particular mean nothing at all.

"Deep cleansing"

This term has always baffled me. How deep is deep? Sounds like a dentist cleaning your teeth. I can vividly hear the sound of the drill trying to get into the skin. If a product could clean deeply—I mean really deeply—it would mean you'd be bleeding. On the other hand, if they figuratively mean *deep clean* to represent a thorough cleansing, that would be fine.

But most women believe that somehow these deep-cleansing products can get into a pore and eject a blackhead. There isn't a product anywhere that can accomplish that. If there were such a product I would have found it, and you would have, too, and neither of us would ever have a problem with blackheads again. No matter how many products I have bought that claimed they could clean out pores, dry up oil, and remove blackheads, they have never once accomplished what they said they could do.

"Famous celebrities like [name of any notable celebrity] are praising this treatment or product."

Somewhere, down deep, many of us have the belief that wherever celebrities flock, particularly when it comes to skin care, that must be where the fountain of youth exists. Nothing could be further from the truth. Just because celebrities can afford to waste their money and spend time seeking out treatments or products does not make the treatments or products legitimate. Next year these same celebrities will be flying off to partake in the next treatment or product developed for the skin because the one from the previous year didn't work.

"Gentle to the skin"

Products that call themselves "gentle to the skin" often cannot substantiate that claim by their ingredients. But that doesn't stop them from slapping that claim on their label. As with the term *hypoallergenic*, there are no guidelines or specifications about what constitutes a *gentle* product. If you don't read the ingredients listing, you won't know that you're buying something that isn't gentle until you put it on your face (and then it's too late).

Why We Believe All This Stuff

Why do we believe all this advertising rhetoric? Why do we believe that wrinkle creams, astringents and expensive skin care routines, or expensive cosmetics will work to make us look younger despite the evidence to the contrary? Why do we continue to believe what the cosmetics companies want us to believe, when time after time independent sources, from dermatologists to consumer reporters (including me), show repeated evidence that these products can't do what they claim? Why, after all this documentation tells us that spending a lot of money on this stuff is a waste, do we continue to buy it? Not only is the testimony overwhelming, but our own rational abilities tell us to stop and think twice. Why don't we? Why are we still willing to buy these products that are supposed to promote a youthful appearance when deep down we probably know better? After all, how many products can make the same promises before we realize that if they all don't work, someone must be lying? Why do we assume the new product is the one that will work? We aren't just being foolish—or are we?

> After all, how many products can make the same promises before we realize that if they all don't work, a lot of people must be lying?

There is much more in our willingness to believe these claims than just foolishness. It is more complicated than that. I believe there are nine extremely compelling reasons why we get taken in time after time by empty, meaningless ads and claims.

Reason #1. For the most part, cosmetics, skin care products, and, more specifically, wrinkle creams, feel good and take very good care of our skin. We all need to clean our face, and many of us have to fight either dry skin, oily skin or combination skin. One way or the other, without skin care products we would be left with more problems than we started with. Soap all by itself, for the majority of women, leaves the face dry and irritated. Even though many toners contain irritants, they take off that last layer of makeup, which can clog pores. Moisturizers (wrinkle creams are, after all, just moisturizers) are an essential part of taking care of dry skin. So the reason we buy the stuff in the first place is because a great number of these products take good care of the skin. They don't perform the miracles they suggest; they aren't worth the big bucks they frequently cost; but, in general, they do take good care of our skin. Coming to terms with what can be done for the skin and what can't (reading the skin care chapter will help quite a bit) will take you a long way from getting seduced by pretty packaging or a convincing sales pitch.

Reason #2. Skin care products often cause skin care complications or do not eliminate the skin problems you bought them for, so you are in constant search for the right products. You believe the right ones for your skin type are out there somewhere. Now if you could only find them. Skin problems are a recurrent headache. It is the rare individual who doesn't have to be concerned with either acne, wrinkles, dry skin, oily skin, irritation, or a combination of them all. Anything but perfect skin seems to be what we all have, but perfect skin is what we are after. Many times skin problems are exacerbated by the very cosmetics we bought to take care of a problem, or the products simply don't help or change anything. This has happened to all of us, but that doesn't mean we give up hope, because eventually we know we will find what we need. That doesn't mean the products we used in the past were bad; we just need to continue the search to find the right ones.

Most women think the major questions to ask about skin are "Which products will be best for my skin," or "Which products work and which ones don't and where do I find them?" The questions themselves show where the problem exists. It is not so much a search for the right product, but for what ingredients should and should not be in the products we are buying. I will go over the do's and don'ts of how to handle skin care problems, but it is essential that you be aware of your skin's limitations and the truth about what skin care ingredients really can do for the face. Once you learn that even with the most expensive products you can overmoisturize the skin while trying to eliminate dryness, irritate the skin in the name of drying up acne, or make oily skin worse by using so-called oil-free moisturizers, you will be way ahead of the game.

Reason #3. Beauty myths die a long hard death. Once we believe something about our skin, it is very hard to change our mind. I will go over many of these myths in this chapter, but some of my favorites are: dry skin wrinkles faster than oily skin; if you tan slowly, you won't damage your skin; cold water closes pores; you can *dry up acne*; don't squeeze a blemish or it will leave a scar; if you don't start using a moisturizer after you turn eighteen you will wrinkle faster than you would if you did; and face creams cannot be used around the eyes and eye creams cannot be used on the face. None of those statements is true; bet you were surprised about at least one or two.

Letting go of myths isn't easy. It takes information, and some of that information is boring and technical. But once you've assimilated some of the basics, none of these other bogus facts will catch you off guard again.

Reason #4. All the ads, brochures, and what the cosmetics salespeople tell us sounds very convincing. Given the amount of money cosmetics companies spend on packaging, promotions, and advertising, it had better look convincing. The glitter and shine at the cosmetics counters may not be gold, but it sure looks like gold. Everything that glitters is not gold, and even if it were, then it wouldn't matter whose product you bought because it would all be gold. Do not be convinced again and again that because something "sounds" good, it is.

Reason #5. It is very difficult to believe that a cosmetics company would want to take advantage of us when it seems that what they are selling is so beautiful and attractive. This desire to trust in a company's higher purpose is part of what we all want to presume. It is tiresome to be constantly cautious about everything. And the spokesmodels look so convincing and sweet; surely they wouldn't lie to us.

Cosmetics companies have one purpose, and that is to sell their cosmetic products. That is their bottom line. Whether or not they do anything else is not as important as that one objective. Many companies do make good products, and there is definitely nothing wrong with selling products. But to assume that a company has a higher purpose and, as a result, some miraculous formula is a poor consumer assumption.

Reason #6. We want to believe that what they tell us is true. It is somehow reassuring to assume that the $50 you just spent is somehow going to erase a few years or lines from your face. Surely all those scientists and dermatologists must have invented something by now.

We also want to believe that there are wrinkle creams that get rid of wrinkles or astringents that close pores or lipsticks that last all day, but it is important to trust our own sense of reality. If there were wrinkle creams, why would any of us have wrinkles? If astringents or toners closed pores, why would any of us have open pores? If lipsticks really did last all day, why would we end up with our lip print on our coffee cup or napkin? It is okay to accept reality, because being realistic will not make you any less beautiful or prevent you from taking good care of your skin.

Reason #7. The cosmetics companies aren't really lying to us. They aren't exactly telling the truth, but even the most extreme ads hedge their promises and claims with vague language that doesn't really say anything specific. When you see an ad for a wrinkle cream that reduces fine lines, restores suppleness, and rejuvenates the skin, you must remember that any moisturizer can make that claim and not be lying. If I took a dead leaf and put some oil and water on it, I would reduce its fine lines, restore some of its suppleness, and temporarily make it look better—until it dried up again. A moisturizer is a moisturizer is a moisturizer. And moisturizers don't do anything permanent.

Reason #8. Salespeople are well trained to sell you their products. They can be very skilled in subtle though effective sales techniques. The best cosmetic sales tactic is to reinforce a woman's insecurity. This emotional battleground is the salesperson's best weapon and the one the consumer is least equipped to avoid or resist.

See if these routines don't feel familiar: 1) The salesperson reminds the consumer that she is not yet as beautiful as she could be because she isn't yet using the salesperson's products. She offers a lipstick and says, "This color would look much better on you." 2) The salesperson helps the consumer notice all the problems her skin is having (after all, she's the expert—she's supposed to notice these problems). She may ask, "Aren't you concerned about how dry your skin is, particularly around your eyes?" 3) The saleswoman suggests that if the woman continues to make the same skin care mistakes over and over, there can be no hope for her face in the future. "You can't start too soon using this product, because it can only get worse if you wait, and then it may be too late to do anything about it."

It is important to know that cosmetics salespeople are not necessarily trained to be skin care or makeup experts; they are trained to sell products. The only way to defend yourself against their sales techniques is with convictions that are not easy for many women. A strong sense of self-esteem and a security in who you are is important in life and at the cosmetics counters. If you are willing to accept the idea of being rescued by the products being sold to you, you are at the mercy of a good sales pitch. You must recognize now that there are no answers inside these glittering, slick boxes and jars—that what you need is information from independent sources (not fashion magazines) that can teach you how to understand your skin.

I admit that I repeatedly come down fairly hard on cosmetics salespeople. It isn't that I haven't met some wonderful cosmetics salespeople, because I have. There have been many times when these remarkable women have given me insights into the cosmetics industry that would have otherwise been impossible for me to obtain. I also would like to acknowledge from experience that, for the most part, particularly at the department store, selling cosmetics is not an easy or lucrative way to earn a living. Unfortunately, I have also had some difficult encounters with cosmetics salespeople. I have listened to and overheard thousands of crazy conversations about skin care and makeup application that are nothing more then sheer sales pressure and incorrect information. Because it is generally hard for the consumer to differentiate between sales technique and valid information, it is my job as a consumer advocate to assume that you are more likely to encounter salesmanship than pure facts. That way you will be prepared no matter what happens when you are shopping for makeup.

Reason #9. This reason is perhaps my most controversial point, but I believe it to be true. As women we have both feminine and masculine parts of our personality. The feminine part is more tolerant, subtle, cooperative, and understanding. The masculine part of our nature is the part of us that is able to be investigative, reactive, assertive, and resolute. It is not natural for many of us to use our masculine nature. Given that the entire issue of beauty and cosmetics in our culture is intrinsically feminine, it definitely is steeped in the most feminine part of our personalities. Perhaps it is our very femininity that keeps us from questioning those things that the salespeople and ads tell us, even when we know they sound farfetched.

Are men less subject to sales pressure than women? Perhaps not. But I would suggest that it is part of a man's feminine nature that makes him less assertive. We all have the capacity to have both masculine and feminine parts to our personality. When we are in the role of consumer, it is to our advantage to be more assertive, particularly at the cosmetics counters, where being feminine is the name of the game.

This last reason of why we tend to believe exaggerated cosmetic claims is perhaps the hardest one to resolve. There is no way I can teach every woman how to ask questions, how to disagree, or how to not believe everything that is being sold to them when it comes to cosmetics. Nor can I make promises about the reaction you will receive when you are no longer yielding and accommodating. My suggestion is to take it one step at a time. Perhaps the next time you are at a cosmetics counter, you can try a few more probing questions and see how the salesperson reacts and how it feels for you to be more assertive. Once you do, it is certain that you will be less likely to leave feeling oversold again. The more information you have, the less susceptible you will be to the hype and fantasy the cosmetics industry confronts us with everywhere we turn.

Whom Should You Believe?

Wouldn't it be easy if the answer were just to believe me and then be done with it? Not that I don't want you to believe what I'm saying, but it is still your job as the cosmetics consumer to figure out exactly what you are going to do about the information you receive, whether it is from me or the cosmetic companies. When it comes to beauty decisions, that is no easy task. There is not much reality or rationality associated with makeup and skin care. Yet without a firm basis in reality and rational thinking, there is no way to approach the cosmetics industry in a reasonable, sober light. What I mean by reasonable and sober is keeping your feet on the ground and your head out of the fluffy sales techniques that accompany cosmetics. It doesn't mean that you can't attain an image of beauty or glamour you're comfortable with; it just means you will do it more easily and with more confidence. Once you take the emphasis off who has the best products and concentrate on what you need to look for in a product that best suits your skin type and personal preferences, there is much you can accomplish and enjoy.

The first battle is trusting what you already know to be true. From mascara to astringents, no cosmetic can do anything earth-shattering for you, no matter whose name is on the label. And one company does not have all the right products for you, because each and every cosmetic line has good and bad products. That doesn't mean there aren't some great products available, because there are, but even great products can have drawbacks. You need to recognize those things if you're going to keep your feet and face firmly planted in looking good and buying wisely.

> Once you take the emphasis off who has the best products and concentrate on what you need to look for in a product that best suits your skin type and personal preferences, there is much you can accomplish and enjoy.

What I mean by facing the "reality" about cosmetics is best illustrated by an example that has nothing to do with cosmetics. I think that shopping for cosmetics is much like shopping for a beautiful pair of shoes. The salesperson brings out this absolutely gorgeous, to-die-for pair of high heels of red Italian leather and studded with multicolored rhinestones that fan out from the pointed toe and continue back to the elegant three-and-a-half-inch heel. Your feet slip into them like Cinderella's foot into the glass slipper. As you turn around in the mirror, admiring the way they look, your entire profile is reflected like something out of a magazine ad. It's amazing what a pair of shoes can do for your appearance.

Unfortunately, the storybook never followed Cinderella home immediately after the ball. We were all told that she ran home at midnight because of her fairy godmother's warning. The truth is, dancing in those glass slippers made her feet swell and ache so much she couldn't wait to get home. The dreamy look in her eyes when she was dancing with the prince wasn't because of the prince, it was from thoughts of soaking her aching corns in hot soapy water. And the slipper she left behind wasn't a mistake, she would have gladly left both of them, but she couldn't get the other one off! Get the picture?

Every time I shop for makeup, do my own makeup, or do someone else's makeup, I try to remember this image. The difference between the way we look without makeup and the way we look when a good makup job is applied is indeed dramatic. I would be the last person to deny the power of beautifully applied makeup. Yet the way we look with makeup on doesn't reflect the effort it takes to apply it, keep the look fresh all day long, or the process of finally washing it off at night. Makeup can make you look great, but that *great look* can represent a lot of effort and bother. Wearing makeup involves some amount of give and take along with the expense. Balancing this give and take means discovering your best cosmetic options based on the most and least of what you can expect from your makeup. This is the real world of cosmetics that I will present to you.

Brand Name Addiction

The question I am asked most frequently is, Which product line do I like the best? Or, What do I think of Lancôme, Estee Lauder, or Nu Skin? That was the major reason I wrote *Don't Go to the Cosmetics Counter Without Me*. By actually reviewing each line, I could point out specifically what we already know is true—that every line, regardless of price, has good and bad products. Brand name loyalty does not make any sense. Lancôme makes a great mascara and some great foundations, but their eyeshadows are too shiny and their oil-free foundation goes on way too thick and heavy. Estee Lauder has some great foundations, a good mascara, and great eye and lip pencils, but the cleanser is too greasy, the foundation colors are oftentimes too pink or orange, and their eye-shadow colors are too shiny or maybe too intense for most women. I could go on and on, but that is basically what happens with every cosmetics line we shop.

The thing is, we already know this one to be true. Yet the success of the major product lines in establishing brand name loyalty is astonishing. It is particularly apparent in how a woman responds to the question about what brand of makeup she is currently using. The answer usually reflects the amount of money she has spent on said product. A customer usually whispers or acts a bit embarrassed when she admits to using a drugstore brand, but if she's using the expensive brand you can hear her across the room. The reality is that the cost of any cosmetic product has nothing to do with whether it will work for you or not. I have used both inexpensive and expensive makeup that looked wonderful and was good for the skin as well as expensive and inexpensive makeup that looked awful and was bad for the skin.

The other point about brand name loyalty is that when we buy a product from a particular cosmetics line, that company is not necessarily manufacturing that product. Many of the eye pencils you are buying from different companies come from the same manufacturer in Germany. Many eyeshadow brands come from the exact same labs. The cosmetics company's main job is to develop the packaging, distribution, and promotion of a product—not always the product itself.

Years ago, just after I opened my first makeup store, I had the opportunity to visit one of the manufacturing plants that was wholesaling their makeup to me. As they proudly showed me around their facilities, showing me the rows and rows of material and machinery, we passed an area where they were assembling eyeshadow tins. At the end of this conveyor were boxes labeled with most of the major cosmetic brand names. They obviously wanted me to know that I would be selling the same stuff these big shots were selling. They were right—I was impressed. I was also pleased to know firsthand how things really happened.

If the notion of one cosmetics company having all the scientific development, particularly that of European scientists, on their side is what keeps you hooked into one line over another, keep in mind that cosmetics chemists change jobs all the time. Get a chance to talk to any one of them and they will tell you how absurd the claims and promises made about the products are.

What I have just described is the reality of the cosmetics industry. I'm hardly the first person to discover this. The television show *60 Minutes* did a segment on this very issue, and Ralph Nader has argued the point himself on numerous talk shows and in his own book on the cosmetics business, as have other consumer reporters. The long and short of it is that no matter who's making your makeup, the end result is that you could get stuck paying a 500 to 2,000 percent markup in what you pay for the final product if you buy according to packaging or advertising claims rather than effect. The package doesn't tell you anything about the product, and the price doesn't reflect anything about the quality—how it will go on the skin or how long the effect you're looking for will last.

Why is it, then, that a particular brand of cosmetics gets to be so expensive when compared to a less expensive brand that has been purchased from the same manufacturing company? In the final analysis, price is determined by what the market will bear. If you're willing to pay twenty-five dollars for a foundation and believe you'll look twenty-five dollars better, they'll sell it to you for just that. Hopefully, by now your ideas of brand name loyalties have changed. Don't take my word for it! Go to any library and check out a copy of *Drug and Cosmetic Industry* magazine and you can read about the manufacturing of cosmetics and cosmetic ingredients. This periodical will reveal how the cosmetics industry works.

When women ask me what I think about a particular brand of cosmetics, my response, regardless of the line, is always the same: there are products in every line that are wonderful, mediocre, awful, or just a total waste of money. The only way to ascertain that is to try the stuff on and see what happens—or read my book *Don't Go to the Cosmetics Counter Without Me*.

Myth Busting

I've been wanting to do this for a long time. The list here is only an overview of what I will explain in more detail later. I just need to let it all out before I go any further, or I will bust. Some of these will shock you and others will come as no surprise, but I can tell you this: each one of these myths that you abandon will save you more money over the years at the cosmetics counter than we both can count.

"Dry skin ages faster than oily skin."

Ah—if that were only true, I would only have to worry about my hair turning gray, but that isn't the case. Dry skin and wrinkling are not associated. They are two distinctly separate skin processes. If dry skin and wrinkling were associated, then ten-year-old kids with dry skin would have wrinkles, and they don't. What we now know is that the sun ages the skin—that almost 90 percent of the wrinkles we see on the skin come from the sun. Dry skin can look more wrinkled while it is dehydrated, but those aren't permanent wrinkles, just dehydrated skin. Slap a little oil and water on the skin (that's what moisturizers in all price ranges are mostly made of) and the skin will look smoother, but you will not have changed a real wrinkle.

"The darker the skin, the tougher it is and less sensitive to irritants than lighter skin."

Nothing could be further from the truth. Skin color has nothing to do with skin sensitivity or skin problems. In fact, African-American women and most women of color can suffer from hyperpigmentation (dark, ashy gray patching) when the skin is even slightly irritated or sun-damaged. There is even some recent scientific evidence that suggests that sun damage may not be determined solely by skin color. There are studies being conducted that seem to indicate that the genetic background of a person and not the skin color is what determines the skin's ability to protect itself from the sun. Dark-skinned women need to protect their skin from the sun as much as light-skinned women.

"Oriental women have perfect skin and rarely have problems."

Oriental women do have fewer problems with enlarged pores or acne than other women do, but they have much greater problems with dry skin and eczema. The skin of Orientals is considered to be more sensitive than most skin types in this regard and more troubled by harsh ingredients. Of course, I would suggest that all skin types are troubled by harsh ingredients, but it may take some time for the cosmetics industry to recognize this basic fact.

"Men's facial skin ages more slowly than that of women."

Something about men shaving and thereby stimulating cell removal and cell growth seems to be the rationale for this very chauvinistic, very erroneous, long-standing myth. Men who shave on a regular basis supposedly increase the skin's natural ability to slough the outer layers of skin. This sloughing action supposedly encourages new cell growth, which is supposed to prevent wrinkles.

First of all, men wrinkle for the same reason women do —exposure to the sun. Second, if shaving did play a role, how would that explain the skin around the eyes and foreheads? Men don't shave their eyes or foreheads, so if shaving had something to do with this cell growth phenomenon, how do men manage to ward off the wrinkles in those areas? Third, sloughing the skin does not necessarily create new skin cells, it just makes room for them. And fourth, even if sloughing the skin did create new skin cells, there is no evidence that doing so can affect wrinkles. The truth is, men who sit in the sun without sun protection get just as many wrinkles as women do. Staying out of the sun—not cell renewal and definitely not shaving—prevents wrinkles. If there is any truth to this notion of men wrinkling less than women, it may have something to do with women being more addicted to the sun than men, thereby damaging their skin through ultraviolet radiation, but that is it.

"Stress ages the skin."

This is a recent myth created by the cosmetics industry. There is no evidence that stress ages the face. The idea is very enticing for a woman living in the nineties. It may seem that stress is aging us, but it has nothing to do with wrinkles. It may have to do with tired bodies and spirits, which may indeed be reflected in the skin, but that still has nothing to do with how the skin ages. The leathery lines we associate with aging come from the sun, plain and simple. Most of the products that advertise themselves as reducing stress on the surface of the skin do not contain ingredients that can live up to the claim. A soothing cleansing treatment and lightweight moisturizer (either expensive or inexpensive) can make the exact same claim.

"Pollution is the skin's new enemy."

If that were true, then women in smog-ridden Los Angeles would be reported as having worse skin than, say, women in Albuquerque or

Portland, and that is not the case. Dermatologists do not see a concentration of skin problems in smog-plagued areas. Skin aging and skin problems seem not to be related to pollution. Pollution particles are simply too large to be absorbed into the skin and cause any permanent damage, plus pollution is washed off at night along with makeup. However, the concept of a cosmetic that promises to keep pollution off the skin is sure to sell lots of products, even though it won't be any different in formulation than any other moisturizer on the market.

"Facial exercises can help eliminate wrinkles."

Many women are under the assumption that skin sags because the muscles in the face become less firm with age. That is not true. Of all the muscles in the body, the facial muscles are most continuously used throughout life. Ninety percent of the wrinkles and sags on the face are there because of sun exposure, not because of sagging facial muscles. If anything, because stretching the skin can be associated with facial lines becoming deeper (notice that laugh lines, the areas of the face we use the most, set in before other lines), overusing the skin by moving it around in the name of strengthening muscles can actually make the skin stretch and sag more.

"Only teenagers get blemishes."

I believed that one for years. Every year I expected my acne to go away and, by the age of twenty-five, when it was still there (and still is), I realized that someone somewhere wasn't telling the truth. The reality is that a large number of women in their twenties to middle thirties get acne. There is also a noticeable increase in acne for women who start experiencing the symptoms of menopause. Teenagers do indeed get acne, and sometimes they outgrow it and sometimes they don't—or sometimes they temporarily outgrow it and then it starts all over again.

"Chocolate causes acne."

Unless you are allergic to chocolate, there is no correlation between chocolate and acne. The same is true for other suspect foods—milk, pizza, fried foods, and anything containing oil. They don't cause acne unless you personally are allergic to them.

"You need specially formulated creams for each part of your body."

Frequently the ingredients in eye creams, throat creams, hand creams, face lotions, and body lotions are the same. There is no reason not to use any one of them wherever you have dry skin.

"Cold water closes pores and hot water opens pores."

Cold water shocks the skin, temporarily swelling it, which makes the pores look smaller for all of about thirty seconds until the skin goes back to its natural state. Hot water burns the skin, irritating the skin and making it swell, which can also break capillaries. Warm water can make the skin softer temporarily because of temporary water retention, but that's about it.

"Do not squeeze blemishes or you will scar."

If you oversqueeze and damage the skin, you can create sores or scabs that can indeed scar the skin. However, if you are careful, squeezing a blemish or a blackhead can be the fastest way to get rid of it.

"All you need is soap to take care of your skin."

In the middle of any discussion about skin care products someone inevitably will say to me, "My mother, who is over seventy, has used only soap or cold cream on her face all her life, and she doesn't have any wrinkles." Whether the skin is wrinkled or not has nothing whatsoever to do with soap or cold cream. Skin care isn't what affects the wrinkling process. Keeping out of the sun or religiously using a strong sunscreen, inheriting good skin, and being healthy (which includes not smoking or frequently losing and gaining weight) are the only ways to prevent the skin from wrinkling and looking aged. If this seventy-year-old woman had been using expensive products, the same claim could be made and the same would be true: skin care doesn't affect the way the skin ages (unless we are talking about the use of sunscreens).

"If you tan slowly, you won't damage your skin."

There is no such thing as a safe tan. Skin that tans will eventually get leathery and run the risk of developing skin cancer.

"Blue eyes are enhanced by blue eyeshadow, and
green eyes are enhanced by green eyeshadow."

There are several problems with this logic: 1) The eye area is too small an area to base an entire makeup scheme upon. 2) What about other factors such as skin, hair, or clothing colors? 3) If the goal is to make blue eyes look bluer, then blue is the wrong color. If you want to make a particular color look more intense, put the opposite color next to it. If you want white to look whiter, you don't put white next to it—you put black next to it. So if your only goal were to make your blue eyes look bluer, you would put orange next to them, not blue—but that wouldn't look very attractive either. The major considerations for choosing eyeshadow will be discussed in the chapters on makeup application.

"Eating more oil will alleviate dry skin."

Drink all the oil you want and if you have dry skin, you will still have dry skin—and a stomachache. Oil on the surface of the skin can prevent dryness.

"Drinking more water will prevent dry skin."

There is a definite benefit to drinking more water, but not for the sake of adding more moisture to the skin. The body can use only the water it needs and the rest is eliminated. Drinking more water will not change your dry skin, but it will change how many trips you make to the bathroom.

"Vitamin E oil rubbed on stretch marks or scars will help get rid of them."

If you rub vitamin E oil, collagen creams, or other emollients over stretch marks and scars, they will not go away. The skin will be less dry, but that won't change a stretch mark or a wrinkle. Both stretch marks and wrinkles are caused by the deterioration of collagen and elastin in the dermis, and creams can't rebuild them.

What the Cosmetics Industry Does Right

As I've admitted before, I know I come down pretty hard on the cosmetics industry, and for some pretty darn good reasons, if I do say so myself. But it would be inappropriate and myopic of me not to mention what the cosmetics companies do right. And they do a lot of things right. I know that sounds ironic, but it is true. Remember, I stated earlier that many of the skin care products and makeup items we buy for the most part do work. They don't all work the same —some work better than others—but for the most part they work pretty well. That isn't accidental. It's the result of a great deal of effort by the industry to make better, more competitive products. Cosmetics chemists do an incredible job of making our cosmetics feel beautiful and look beautiful, and I don't sing their praises often enough.

What the cosmetics industry is doing right is making cosmetics better and better. Almost all types of cosmetics have improved over the years. How the products feel and how they work on the skin have come a long way since the sixties and seventies—particularly in the case of moisturizers. A lot of effort is being exerted to make lotions that keep moisture in the skin for longer periods of time. There are many new technical devices that help a cosmetics chemist know how well a product is working on the skin. Some of these tests, such as computer-enhanced image analysis of the skin, measuring the skin's water loss, measuring the elasticity of the skin, and measuring the skin's texture, are currently being used to look at product effectiveness.

Of course, the claims about the test results from these procedures are still exaggerated. What these tests reveal is rarely noticeable to the human eye. Plus, we are still only talking about water retention, not the elimination of wrinkles. Overrated as these new skin tests are, however, they still give the chemist a more systematic process than mere guesswork to evaluate a product.

There are also new ingredients that can help the skin stay moist with fewer pores getting blocked. Liposomes, collagen, hyaluronic acid, glycols, mucopolysaccharides, sodium PCA, allantoin, amino acids, cholesterol, fatty acids, and elastin are just a few of the new ingredients that can retain, bind, and hold water in the skin. The benefits of these ingredients for the consumer can be quite good. Again, we are not talking miracles, just improved quality of some skin care products.

As you may have already expected to hear, there is a hitch to all this. Most of the fancy testing is being done for skin care products, mainly moisturizers and so-called wrinkle creams. The area of formulation that still leaves much to be desired is makeup products. I often wonder when the cosmetics industry will start using feedback from the consumer to make decisions about lipstick, foundation, or mascara formulations.

Chapter Two
Finding the Best Skin Care
Routine Possible

Why Does It Have to Be So Complicated?

As I look over the material and research I've accumulated, from magazine articles, books, and medical reviews to interviews with dermatologists and cosmetics chemists, it seems amazing to me that I've been able to sort through it all. You wouldn't think that cleansing the face, moisturizing the skin, and fighting blemishes could be so complicated or shrouded in such controversy, but it certainly is. Perhaps an explanation for the complicated array of information is the very nature of the skin and our intense feelings about how we look.

The face, even though it occupies such a small surface area of the body, manifests a lot of topical problems: acne, wrinkles, sagging skin, sunburn, blackheads, dryness, irritation, eczema, and allergies, not to mention our very notions of what beauty is all about. And there is a lot of money to be made if you can get a consumer to believe that your products will work for her.

No wonder it's so complicated and hard to decipher. My job now is to present all this information in a way that helps you understand your skin and what it does and doesn't need so you find a good cleansing routine and can stop wasting money on useless cosmetic products.

> The odds are that you will eventually be one of those women who change their skin care routine every three years and try something new.

Before I do any of that, let me mention my major philosophy about skin care products and the skin care routine you are presently using. If the products you are currently using work for you, no matter how expensive or inexpensive, and you are satisfied with how your skin looks and feels, continue doing exactly what you are doing. If you feel you aren't spending too much money and all the products make you and your skin happy, there is absolutely no reason in the world to change. I don't want someone to use a new routine, mine or anyone else's, unless she is dissatisfied with what she is now doing!

My ideas and suggestions present options and alternatives. There is no reason to change just for the sake of change. Statistics indicate that most women who buy cosmetics change their cleansing routine or moisturizer every three years. The odds are that you will eventually be one of those women who change their skin care routine and try something new. What you are about to read could change the way you spend money on skin care the next time you're ready to make a change. Without question, my suggestions about skin care can save you hundreds, if not thousands, of dollars over the years. My skin care routine for all skin types is famous for costing about $15. (It used to cost $10, but times have changed.) When you do decide to do something different for your skin, these ideas will still be valid. I've been following my own advice for almost fourteen years now.

I should also mention that my ideas are somewhat radical in comparison to those of most "beauty" experts on both sides of the counter. I am known for being a proponent of good skin care that results in beautiful skin but does not take a lot of time and does not consume my life. I do not want to be preoccupied with my skin for fifteen minutes every morning and evening, with an hour-long weekend ritual thrown in for good measure. There are two reasons why I feel so strongly about this. The first one is that most women don't have the time to bother (I barely have the time to eat dinner, much less waste time with elaborate skin care routines); and second and most important, the extra time will not make a difference in the way your skin will look anyway. If I had evidence that the extra products and the extra skin cleansing and masking time made a difference in the way skin looked, I would be the first one to find the time to make it happen. But there is nothing in a complicated skin care routine that makes it any more effective than a simple one. I will prove that as I explain how to take care of your skin.

The other thing that makes my viewpoint on cleansers, soaps, astringents, toners, and facial masks controversial are the products I *don't* recommend. I am frustrated by most experts continuing to recommend products I find irritating and painful to the skin. Regardless of whether they are recommending natural products, instant youth products, or consumer products, their recommendations all sound the same to me. These experts still counsel women with oily skin to use alcohol-based toners, soaps that are too drying, scrubs that are too abrasive, facial masks that aggravate the skin, or combinations of those things, which are too much for anyone's skin to handle. For women with dry or mature skin, there are still the endorsements for eye creams, cell-renewal creams, and so-called special night creams or day creams. But I'll get to all of that in the next few pages, too. The point I want to make here is that if my ideas sound different, it's because they are. I'll do my best to explain why I feel this way, and you can then figure out what you as the consumer want to do about it.

The Skin Care Routine Everyone Should Avoid

Before I delve further into the specifics of my skin care routine, I'd like to describe what happens when you follow the typical skin care routine recommended for many women by many of the major cosmetic companies. Product specifics can vary from company to company, but the basic routine is more or less the same (you'll recognize it immediately). Remember, the following is what you should *not* do.

First, you wipe off your makeup with a water-soluble cleanser that makes your face feel greasy or dry depending on which one you use. Following the cleanser, you apply an alcohol-based toner or astringent to remove any remaining cleanser, and this makes the face feel dry. Now the problem of dry skin is met by the moisturizer, which undoes the previous step of using a toner. Now that you are cleansed, toned, and moisturized, you can finally apply your makeup. After you get your makeup on, you're then told to use face powder to reduce the shine caused by the moisturizer you just put on. Now that you're not shining anymore (heaven forbid you should shine), you are sold iridescent eyeshadows, iridescent blushes, and shiny lip glosses so you can shine all over again. Get the picture?

In all fairness to the cosmetics companies, there are cleansers available that rinse off clean without using a washcloth; there are toners that don't contain alcohol (or other irritants); and most moisturizers take very good care of dry skin. It isn't those products I take issue with. There are just too many of you who spend a lot of money on the skin care routine I described above and don't understand why you have dry, irritated, oily skin all at the same time. My job is to help you to find those products that can keep this from happening to you again. They're out there; you just have to know what to look for and why.

Searching for Your Skin Type!

I've been promising to shake up your long-standing beliefs about skin care, so I might as well start at the beginning with figuring out your skin type. Beauty experts and cosmetics salespeople have been struggling with skin type for a long time. In my opinion, it is one of the most misleading and misused beauty concepts around, and it is usually how we begin making decisions about our skin care routines.

Regardless of how sophisticated some companies are in approaching the issue, using computers or questionnaires to help you discover what is going on with your skin, the way the final determination for skin type is made is usually inaccurate. That's not to say that understanding skin type isn't important; it's just not the way the cosmetics industry approaches it or the way we've been indoctrinated to think about it.

The first problem with knowing your skin type is that you can't know what type of skin you have before you evaluate what you're currently doing to clean your face. How you clean your face can affect its oiliness, dryness, or sensitivity and it can aggravate an acne flare-up. The skin type your face feels like right now is primarily (although not solely) a result of the way you clean your face. Your skin care routine can be creating the very problems you're trying to eliminate. For example, if you wash every day with a bar soap (which is drying) and then follow up with a moisturizer (which can be greasy and potentially can block pores), you can create a severe combination skin condition. Or if you wipe off your makeup with a cream (which is greasy), then follow up with a toner (which is drying), you should not be surprised if you develop a combination skin condition accompanied by dry patches and breakouts. Or if you have a normal skin type and use an alcohol-based toner and scrub, you can find your skin very dry. Typing skin without taking into consideration what you now use assumes that the skin is the way it is all by itself, regardless of what you do to it, and that is not always the case. Before you can know what your skin type really is, sometimes you have to start back at square one to discover what your skin type is *not*.

The second problem with discovering your skin type is the notion that once you've been typed, your skin will stay the same forever, or at least until you grow older, and that isn't necessarily true either. Day to day, month to month, and season to season, the face is subject to emotions, weather conditions, menstrual cycles, and whatever else life brings with it. All these things can directly affect skin type. If your skin care routine focuses on skin type, then your routine becomes obsolete the moment the season changes or you decide to change boyfriends. What do you do then— run out and buy new products? If you go to the cosmetics counter today and the salesperson determines your skin type, she can only base that judgment on what your skin feels and looks like at that moment. If she then makes a decision about what products you should use based only on that information, she is making a big mistake.

I can't tell you how many women I've met who get one blemish and run to the dermatologist complaining about acne. Or the women who start seeing a line or two appear around their eyes and immediately buy the most expensive eye cream they can find.

The third reason that the concept of skin type can be misleading or misused is that some women frequently find themselves with all skin types! Over the years, even when using gentle, irritant-free products, I've experienced irritated skin patches at the same time I had oily skin, an acne flare-up, and dry skin around my eyes. Present that list to cosmetics salespeople and they go wild. If I followed what they told me at the cosmetics counter I would have to buy a little bit of everything to handle all these problems. And it is not an unusual problem for women to have a little bit of each skin type going on simultaneously or overlapping each other.

The fourth problem with identifying skin type is the way the cosmetics industry handles that information. The idea promoted by the cosmetics industry is that every woman can and should have normal skin. The very idea of normal skin is a slippery issue. Like the rest of our bodies, skin is in a constant state of change. Even women with perfect complexions will go through phases of having oily or dry skin. They may even have breakouts once in a while. Given that skin is so volatile, no one is likely to have normal skin for very long, no matter what she does. Those of us who don't have normal skin and instead struggle with oily skin, breakouts, dry skin, or sensitive skin know that normal skin is at best elusive. If finding your skin type helps you control your skin problems better, that's great, but if it sets you up to lust after normal skin, don't hold your breath.

The fifth problem with determining skin type is that it is highly subjective, and this one has little to do with the cosmetics industry. Most women really do have wonderful skin but refuse to accept it. They are distressed by the smallest blemish, wrinkle, or slightest sensation of dry skin. I can't tell you how many women I've met who get one blemish and run to the dermatologist complaining about acne. Or the women who start seeing a line or two appear around their eyes and immediately buy the most expensive eye cream they can find in the hope of warding off their worst imagined nightmare. Overreacting to what you see in the mirror makes for more mistakes in cosmetics purchases than almost any other aspect of skin type. This is one of those times where being realistic is the most important part of your skin care routine.

The sixth problem with identifying your skin type involves the ubiquitous combination-skin complaint. The puzzle is that almost everyone at some time or another, if not all the time, has combination skin. Which is not surprising; that happens to be the way the skin functions. The nose, chin, center of the forehead, and center of the cheek areas have more oil glands than other parts of the face, and so it is not surprising to discover that those areas tend to be oilier and to break out more than the other areas of the face. To call combination skin a special skin type is almost unnecessary because so many women have it. Problems occur when you start segmenting the face and buying two sets of products—those to deal with the oily areas and those to deal with the dry areas—or buying products that are supposedly designed for combination skin because they contain different ingredients, when they rarely do. Combination skin does not mean you need two sets of skin care products or that you need to do dra-matically different things to the different areas of your skin. Products designed for combination skin can actually make the condition worse.

The last problem and the most frustrating one is that skin type is often used (by cosmetics salespeople and the cosmetics industry in their ads) to instigate a sense of inferiority and helplessness when shopping for skin care products. Once your skin is a "type" and it isn't normal, a sense of desperation can set in. (Or if it is normal, then you had better do what you can now to make sure it stays that way.) I've seen it happen a thousand times over as I've listened to or been subjected to the salesperson's kind rebuke about the mistakes a woman is making for her particular skin type (which mostly has to do with the fact that she's not using the products being sold at that particular counter). Skin type is not a death sentence that is then vindicated by the products you buy. Having a particular skin type does not mean your skin will fall off or that you will wrinkle any faster or a less beautiful woman because of it. Skin type is not cured by cosmetic products; yes, it can be controlled or alleviated, but it can't be cured. Skin type is a direction or an indicator of the type of products you should be using, and that is all. Do not make it any more or less than that.

Summary:

1 Your real skin type can be camouflaged by the skin care products you are now using. Skin can be made dry by products that contain alcohol; oily skin can be made oilier by being over-irritated with scrubs and harsh ingredients; and mature skin can be made to look dull by using rich moisturizers that are too greasy.

2 Skin type changes with emotions, weather conditions, and menstrual cycles. You need to recognize these changes when they happen and adapt your skin care routine accordingly. That

doesn't mean running out and buying new products; it may only require cutting back on one step of your cleansing routine or increasing another.

3 Sometimes women find that their faces exhibit more than one skin type simultaneously. When more than one skin type is present, it doesn't necessarily mean more products are needed; it may mean being more gentle with your skin so you don't aggravate the condition further or using a lighter moisturizer that doesn't clog pores.

4 The idea of identifying your skin type so that you can make it "normal" is not realistic. The goal can't be that everyone will have normal skin. The goal is to have as smooth a skin as is possible for your skin type. There are ways to achieve that, but hoping for normal skin will only frustrate your efforts and waste your money.

5 Skin type is highly subjective. What may look like normal skin to one person may seem oily or wrinkled to another. The cosmetics industry racks up most of its sales on your unjustifiably low self-esteem and insecurity.

6 To call combination skin a special skin type separate from oily or dry skin is almost unnecessary because most women have it. But that doesn't mean everyone should rush out and buy oily products for dry patches and dry products for oily patches.

7 Skin type should not be used as a tool to beat up your ego. Skin type is only an indicator of the basic type of products and ingredients you should be focusing on. You don't need an entirely different set of products for each skin type, only a different combination of products or a different frequency of use.

Do all these problems mean you can't judge your skin type? Of course not. It just means you need to be careful about what you do with information you receive and be realistic about how you assess your skin type. I've included several categories in addition to the standard skin type lists you are used to seeing. My feeling is that the usual four categories of skin type—dry, oily, mature, and combination—are too general and practically useless for a vast number of women. They never take into account that mature skin is not a type unto itself and that oily skin doesn't necessarily break out and that there isn't only one type of normal skin. The following is my list, which hopefully takes into account all skin types.

You don't need an entirely different set of products for each skin type, only a different combination of products or a different frequency of use.

Basic normal skin. No visible pores; little to no dry skin; few to no breakouts; no excess oil to speak of; no skin sensitivities or allergies present. Depending on sun exposure and skin color, wrinkles may begin to appear between ages thirty-two and thirty-five. (Please note that, despite what the cosmetics industry would like you to believe, *normal* skin does not mean *flawless* skin.)

Mature normal skin. No visible pores; minimal amount of dry skin; eye puffiness on occasion; no excess oil present; minimal presence of whiteheads. Depending on sun exposure and skin color, there can be pronounced wrinkling on the face for women over the age of forty-five.

Basic oily skin. Visible pores; visible blackheads; small breakouts mostly occurring around the nose, cheeks, chin, and forehead. There is a buildup of excess oil that gets worse as the day goes on. Depending on sun exposure and skin color, wrinkles may begin to appear between ages thirty-two and thirty-five. (Please remember that having oily skin does not prevent or slow down wrinkling. Keeping the sun off the face is what prevents or slows down the wrinkling process.)

Severe oily skin. Enlarged pores and blackheads tend to occur over much of the face but are most prominent around the nose, center of the forehead, and cheeks (or T-zone). Excess oil is present almost immediately after washing the face; makeup seems to slide off by the end of the day; there can be intense breakouts during the menstrual cycle or for any reason at all. Depending on sun exposure and skin color, wrinkles may begin to appear between ages thirty-two and thirty-five.

Mature oily skin. Visible pores, blackheads, and a small number of breakouts occur around the T-zone and eye area. Some whiteheads can also be present. Skin around the eyes may be dry and a buildup of excess oil is still noticeable by the end of the day. Makeup seems not to last and skin color can appear dull. Depending on sun exposure and skin color, there can be pronounced wrinkling for women over the age of forty-five.

Acned oily skin. Similar to severe oily skin except that breakouts are more chronic and intense. Blemishes can often leave minor scarring or discoloration. Depending on sun exposure and skin color, wrinkles may begin to appear between ages thirty-two and thirty-five. (This is my skin type.)

Acned dry skin. This is an unusual skin type, but it does exist. Chronic blemishes occur and yet the skin is dry, flaky, and taut, with little or no oil present except a slight amount in the T-zone.

Cystic acne. This type of acne may or may not be accompanied by oily skin. It is distinguished from the mild acne associated with most oily skin types by the large, deep, and disfiguring lesions on the face.

Basic dry skin. No visible pores; skin tends to flake and peel; dry patches are present; lips may feel parched. As the day goes on, the skin tends to feel more dry and tight. Depending on sun exposure and skin color, wrinkles may begin to appear between ages thirty-two and thirty-five.

Mature dry skin. No visible pores; skin tends to flake and peel; dry patches are present; lips may feel very dry and actually crack. As the day goes by, the skin can feel very dry and tight. There can also be a "dull" appearance to the surface of the skin from a lack of natural color. Depending on sun exposure and skin color, there can be pronounced wrinkling between ages forty-five and fifty.

Sensitive skin. Regardless of the presence of any other skin type, your skin tends to react to everything you put on it and to your emotions. The reaction can be in the form of blemishes, dry patches, redness, irritation, puffy eyes, dry lips, and/or dry skin.

Combination skin. The presence of any two of the above skin types occurring simultaneously.

Summary:

All of these skin types exist, but they can be affected to a large extent by your present skin care routine and the weather, as well as your diet, emotions, and makeup routine. No skin type falls exclusively into one category or the other. Frequently, more than one skin condition is present at the same time. The advertising gimmick of normal skin is a frustrating myth that is more like the proverbial carrot in front of the horse—always there, never to be reached. Because of that passionate search to achieve perfect skin, we end up doing and spending too much for too little return, and often we make the skin condition we are trying to soothe worse.

One more comment. Having come to the point in my life where my skin is entering the category of "mature," I want to explain that *mature* skin does not refer simply to skin with wrinkles—wrinkles have nothing to do with age and everything to do with the sun. But the longer you've spent in the sun the more severe damage can be seen in *mature* skin. If you have not exposed your face to the sun, *mature* skin is skin that has changed in surface appearance due to the genetically controlled slowdown in the rate of cell turnover (see the section on cellular renewal, page 56, for further explanation), which can make skin thinner, drier, and less elastic. How can you tell if you have mature skin? Check out the section on the differences between genetic aging versus photoaging, page 71, for a detailed explanation. The other categories of skin type—everything from oily skin to acned—are not automatically affected by age. "Mature" does not mean your skin won't exhibit blemishes or acne, oiliness, lines, or large pores. There are changes that take place as we mature, but these changes depend on a lot of factors, of which age is only one.

Almost Everyone Has Sensitive Skin

Most of us have sensitive skin. Regardless of your primary skin type, myriad minor (or major) irritating skin conditions can be present. The skin can burn, chafe, and crack, and you may have patchy areas of dry, flaky skin. Skin can also break out in small bumps that look like diaper rash. It can itch, swell, blotch, and redden, and may develop allergic reactions to cosmetics, animals, dust, or pollen. Most of us have sensitive skin to one degree or another because skin is an extremely sensitive body organ.

Your skin is the protective armor that keeps the elements and other invaders from entering the body. We protect most of our anatomy with clothing, but our faces are left painfully exposed to everything. It's no wonder the skin on our faces acts up at least now and then. Sensitive skin is probably the most "normal" type of skin there is.

Most skin care routines separate what they recommend for women with sensitive skin types from what they recommend for women with other skin types. One of the reasons I want you not to overweigh the importance of an individual skin type is that I believe everybody has the potential to develop sensitive skin. Therefore the same precaution taken for sensitive skin affects every skin type. What is that precaution? Treating all skin types gently. Whether you think of your face as oily, dry, or mature, you still need to be gentle with your skin.

The operative word for the rest of this book is *gentle*. Not irritating the skin, regardless of skin type, will be a recurrent theme throughout. Of course, some oily skin can tolerate more than dry skin can, so where differences exist they will be boldly pointed out. But for the most part, if something is bad for sensitive skin, it is probably bad for oily skin, acned skin, dry skin, and mature skin. As you use this information on gentle skin treatment, you will slowly solve skin problems you may have been experiencing.

As you have already realized by now, treating all skin types as gently as possible is one of the many ways my skin care recommendations differ from those of most beauty experts. Because I believe skin care routines have some basic commonalities, I will go over the reasons for and the basic requirements of each step of the cleansing process before I discuss specific recommendations for each skin type. But first you must understand why I am so adamant about being gentle to the skin.

The Skin's Worst Enemies Besides the Sun

There are two external factors that contribute negatively to the health and appearance of the skin: inflammation and irritation. These wreak the most havoc on our skin, and that goes for all skin types. Although many things can cause inflammation and irritation, there is little or no difference in what each can do to the skin. The reason is that skin can't tell the difference between irritation and inflammation, much less pain, itching, or swelling; as far as the skin is concerned, it is all basically the same thing. The skin can handle only so much irritation and inflammation before it reacts adversely. And when the skin reacts, it really reacts. What can happen is an assortment of problems that is hard to combat: redness, dry patches, blemishes, rashes, cracks along the sides of the nose and corners of the mouth and eyes, flakiness, and an increased sensation of sensitivity.

Note: *It is generally believed that irritation and inflammation are not responsible for wrinkles and premature aging of the skin. Some dermatologists suggest, however, that repeatedly using irritating ingredients on sensitive skin areas such as the eyes can make wrinkles worse. Likewise, it is thought that irritation and inflammation can make wrinkles worse. Products that are advertised as making the skin look younger when placed over the lines on the face often contain irritating ingredients (such as alcohol) that swell the skin temporarily. It would seem that with repeated use, they could make the skin more wrinkled.*

Always treat your skin gently or it will complain. The skin may react to topical irritation immediately or it may take some time, but irritate the skin and it will eventually react.

What physically takes place when the skin is irritated? The skin's nerve endings become immediately overstimulated. This stimulation then triggers the nerve endings to stimulate whatever they are attached to. The nerves on the face are attached to the skin, hair follicles, oil glands, capillaries (blood flow to the skin's surface), and the underlying structure of the skin. If you overactivate the nerve endings, the oil glands will produce more oil, the skin will flake, and the blood circulation to the small capillaries near the surface of the skin will increase and possibly cause spiderlike veins to appear. If surface capillaries are already present on your face, irritation will make them worse. Irritate the skin and you end up with more trouble than you bargained for.

It logically follows that learning how to be gentle to your face is one of the most important parts of any skin care routine. There is no way you can ever begin to hope for soft, smooth skin when the face is being irritated every time you cleanse it. Irritation-free skin is the goal. I am going to help you eliminate those things that hurt the face due to irritation.

What You Can Do to Protect Your Skin

There are plenty of emotional and environmental stresses that bombard your skin all the time. Some you can control, and some are much more difficult to control—intense work schedules, a frenzied home life, paying bills, or your car breaking down are all potential problems for the skin. Heat in summer (or in a sauna), cold in winter, sun, wind, and pollution are all forceful drying agents for the face. Many skin care companies would suggest that they can reduce the effects of these external skin bullies with the products in their line. Sometimes they can. Moisturizers will counteract the drying effect of outside cold and inside dry heat during the winter. During the summer a sunscreen with an SPF of 15 or greater can keep the sun off the face and prevent premature wrinkling. Other than sunscreens and moisturizers that prevent dryness, there are no products out there that can reduce the effects of emotional stress on our face or form a force field over the face and keep environmental enemies off our skin. By the way, during the winter, a humidifier in your room or home can go a long way toward reducing dry skin problems.

Separate from the irritants in the environment that confront our skin every day, there are the many things we do to our skin or buy in the way of skin care products that cause even more irritation. Believe me, it is easier to eliminate skin "care" culprits that irritate and inflame our skin than it is to control the environment or our emotional life. With that in mind, here is a list of typical skin care and makeup ingredients and specific cosmetic products to avoid. The skin can react negatively to all of the following products and ingredients.

Irritating Products

abrasive scrubs
astringents containing irritating ingredients
scrub puffs
cold water
facial masks containing irritating ingredients
fresheners containing irritating ingredients
hot water
loofahs

soaps
toners containing irritating ingredients
washcloths

Irritating Ingredients

acetone
alcohol (SD alcohol followed by a number only)
ammonia
ammonium lauryl sulfate (if it is listed first on the label)
avocado (which is very acidic and can burn the skin)
benzoyl peroxide
boric acid
camphor
citrus juices (such as grapefruit or orange)
eucalyptus
menthol
mint
phenol
salicylic acid
sodium lauryl sulfate (if it is listed first on the ingredient label)
witch hazel

These ingredients are more common than you can imagine and they are particularly recommended for women with oily or acned skin. That makes no sense to me, because these ingredients can aggravate oily skin and make acned skin look redder than it already is. Ingredients like camphor, menthol, mint, alcohol, and phenol are sometimes recommended because they are considered to be anti-itch ingredients. The theory works like this: when your skin itches, the nerve endings are sending messages begging you to scratch. If you place these irritating ingredients over the area that itches, the nerve hears the irritation message louder than it hears the itch message and interprets this as a reason to stop itching. That reasoning is all fine and good if minor, occasional itching is your problem. If it is not and those ingredients are used in skin care products meant to be used every day, they can dry out the skin, create rashes, produce more oil, and cause redness. None of those side effects is attractive on the face.

Summary:

Think gentle! What makes my skin care routine different from most others on the market is the theory that the skin doesn't have to hurt or tingle even a little to be clean. (If the skin tingles, it is being irritated, not cleaned.) The major rule for all skin types is, if it irritates the skin, don't do it again. Pain and cleanliness have nothing to do with each other.

Note: *It goes without saying, though I'll say it anyway, that my feelings about the ingredients and products I suggest you avoid are not widely shared by the cosmetics industry as well as some dermatologists and pharmaceutical companies. Although most would agree that these ingredients can irritate the skin, they would argue that the concentrations of these chemicals are so low that the irritation is minimal, or they would assert that some irritation for some skin types is beneficial. I would argue that a lot of people react to "minimal concentrations" of irritating ingredients. Frequently these irritating ingredients are among the first listed on the label, which means they are probably not minimal. Too much irritation is rarely beneficial and it causes more problems than it solves. However, if you use products that contain irritating ingredients and you are not experiencing skin irritation or any other side effects, then you must have exceptionally durable skin. Nevertheless, I would still recommend that you treat it gently, because repeated irritation can eventually catch up with you.*

Cleaning the Face—The First Step

Whether it involves taking off your makeup or cleaning your face when you wake up in the morning, the first order of skin care is washing the face. Notice that I said *washing*—not wiping off or scrubbing, but washing. There is never a time when I recommend that anyone should wipe at her skin or her eyes to get makeup off or to clean the face in the morning. Now how's that for something different?

The cleansing routine I recommend starts with water. The most important part of cleaning your face is using water. That's right, good old-fashioned H_2O. Not water by itself, of course, but I'll soon tell you what you use with the water. Let me tell you why water is so important.

1 Water is an integral part of the human system. Water is compatible with everyone's skin. Wait, I take that back. I've learned over the years never to say never and never to say everyone. There are indeed those people who find even water irritating to the skin, but that is a condition to be dealt with by a dermatologist and not by this book.

2 Water is the most gentle way to clean the face. But water in and of itself is not automatically gentle. Water is only gentle when it is tepid. Hot water can burn and irritate the skin, and

cold water will shock and irritate the skin. If the goal is to be gentle (and it is), then tepid water is essential.

3 Water is frictionless, and this is a very important reason to use water. When you splash your face with water, your hands glide over the face and, yes, prevent you from pulling the skin. That means you can remove your makeup without tugging at your face. This can prevent irritation and reduce some amount of skin sagging. Constantly wiping, tugging, and pulling on the skin, particularly in the eye area, stretches out some of the skin's inherent elasticity. Like a rubber band, the skin can only take so much pulling till it won't snap back anymore.

As essential as water is to any cleansing routine, water alone is not enough. Water by itself will not remove the oil from the skin or your makeup. Even when your makeup is predominantly water soluble, after a long day of wear, mixed with your own oil, perspiration, and favorite moisturizer, it is no longer 100 percent water soluble. To thoroughly clean the face, you need something along with the water that will cut through the makeup and the oil but at the same time be gentle and glide over the skin.

What Type of Cleanser?

All of us are familiar with the three primary categories of cleansers available: wipe-off cleansers (including cold creams and liquid makeup removers), soaps of all kinds, and water-soluble cleansers (creamy, lotion-type cleansers that rinse off). My preference—and this one hasn't changed for years—are water-soluble cleansers.

A good water-soluble cleanser is a terrific invention. It is a cross between a shampoo and a cold cream, and it is not a soap. What differentiates a good water-soluble cleanser from a poor one is that it washes off the makeup without leaving the face dry (like some soap) or greasy (like cold cream); contains no fragrance, coloring agents, or abrasive particles; and most important of all, it is gentle to the skin. There are cleansers on the market that call themselves water soluble, but in actuality they need to be wiped off with a wet washcloth. Whether the cleanser is wiped off dry with a tissue or wet with a washcloth, it is anything but water soluble. Water-soluble cleansers replace the cold-cream-type products that need to be wiped off the skin.

Water-soluble cleansers can be a gentle, efficient way to remove makeup and clean the skin. Everything is done at the sink. Even a heavy makeup wearer can take off all her makeup this way. Using a water-soluble cleanser eliminates the need for a separate eye makeup remover or boxes of tissues to wipe the face with. Imagine splashing your face generously with (tepid) water, then massaging a water-soluble cleanser evenly over your face, including the eyes, and then rinsing it off with more water, preferably with your hands. Once the face is rinsed, it shouldn't feel greasy or dry. It is much more preferable to spreading greasy, oily creams over the face and eyes and then wiping and rewiping them off with tissue or cloths. Doesn't that sound messy and inconvenient? It is.

But not all water-soluble cleansers are created equal, and finding a good one can be tricky. Just because a cleanser is called water soluble doesn't mean it really comes off with water or is gentle. They all have names like Milky or Creamy or Foaming Face Wash or Gel Cleanser that sound great. But many of the cleansers that claim they rinse off leave the face feeling greasy and need to be wiped off, or they rinse off too well, leaving the face feeling dry and irritated.

Case in point: A recent infomercial for cosmetics being sold by Victoria Principal has her sitting in front of a sink, "washing" her face with a supposedly water-soluble cleanser. She delicately taps her face with water as if the water is being rationed and then takes the creamy cleanser and spreads it around her face, rubbing it into her makeup and neck. She then proceeds to take a washcloth and wipe off her makeup. As she is wiping off her makeup she exclaims about how well her makeup is coming off. Of course, it isn't coming off well at all; she is pulling and wiping it off with a washcloth, doing extra tugging around her eyes and eyelashes to get the eye makeup and cleanser off. (When she's done, the washcloth looks fairly murky.) The clincher comes at the end of this demonstration when Victoria applies a pink (containing far too much dye) eye cream by daintily tapping around her eyes, exclaiming that you need to be so careful with the skin in this area. Did she think we didn't see her pulling and tugging at her skin seconds before when she was wiping off her cleanser?

Using washcloths with water to remove your cleanser is not what I'm referring to when I say a product is water soluble. Water-soluble cleansers should splash off without the aid of a washcloth, or if you prefer to use something besides your hands, use a smooth sponge or any smooth cloth. Washcloths are irritating. Many people use smoother cloths on their kitchen counters than they do on their face. Heavy wiping at the face, particularly the eyes, can sag it. It is that simple.

Over the years I have found one cleanser that meets all my requirements and is reasonably priced. I am still recommending Cetaphil Lotion from Owen/Galderma Laboratories. Cetaphil has all the things I look for in a water-soluble cleanser: it is fragrance free, has no coloring agents, is relatively inexpensive and remarkably gentle, and it removes all makeup, including eye makeup. You can find it in most drugstores across the country and around the world in the pharmacy section. There are few other cleansers available that can do what Cetaphil Lotion can. Revlon makes Clean and Clear for Sensitive Skin, but I find it leaves the skin slightly drier than Cetaphil does, though it is an option. Also, La Prairie, for $45, makes a water-soluble cleanser that leaves the skin feeling very good, but not any better than the Cetaphil does (and the price difference is almost $38).

I should mention that there are many water-soluble cleansers on the market that I am a bit reluctant to recommend, but they are worth a shot for some women who suffer from very oily skin. These are a group of water-soluble cleansers that lather up and can leave the skin on the dry side, but they are not as drying as some soaps can be, nor are they in the least bit greasy. (Some women with oily skin may find Cetaphil Lotion a bit too "slippery" feeling on the skin to be comfortable using it, and makeup on oily skin can be more stubborn to remove than it is for other skin types.) L'Oréal makes a cleanser called Active Cleansing Gel; there is another one called Eucerin Foaming Face Wash, and Neutrogena has its Facial Cleansing Formula. All of these can be used at night to remove all your makeup. However, if you find these cleansers to be too drying or irritating over the eye area, I would strongly suggest first going over the eye area with Cetaphil Lotion to remove the eye makeup, then finishing with one of these other cleansers. In the morning I would again recommend using Cetaphil Lotion. With Cetaphil Lotion most skin types, specifically normal and oily skin types, won't need to be moisturized, because the lotion doesn't leave your face dry after it is washed off. But more about that later.

Reminder: *Do not use specialty eye-makeup removers, and avoid all cleansers that need to be wiped off with either tissues, cotton balls, or washcloths.*

Summary:

Water-soluble cleansers, which rinse off completely when water is splashed on the face and leave the face feeling clean but not dry or greasy, are the best and most convenient way to clean the face. Creamy-type cleansers, especially when it is recommended that they be removed with a washcloth, pull at the skin and can sag it. There are many types of water-soluble cleansers on the market, so you have to be careful when choosing one for your skin. Many foaming or gel-type cleansers are indeed water soluble, but they may contain ingredients that can be drying or irritating to the face and eyes.

Basic Directions: *Wash your hands first and then splash the face generously with tepid water (not hot or cold). Once the face is soaking wet, take your cleanser and massage it generously all over the face, including the eyelids. Rinse very well. If there are traces of makeup left behind, repeat this step one more time. Another option is to first cleanse the eye area and rinse; then do the rest of the face separately and rinse again. This step is done twice a day or whenever you need to clean the face, whether or not you are wearing makeup.*

What About Bar Soap?

Those of you who are familiar with the other editions of *Blue Eyeshadow* already know I am not thrilled with bar soap. But given the popularity of its use, it requires more description than I've given it in the past. Before, I would have said absolutely no bar soap! There are problems with using most bar soaps no matter what type of skin you have. Actually, I don't have to tell you that, because those of you who have used bar soap—and most of you have—already know it can dry and irritate the skin. But there still might be a selection of soaps available that some women may be able to use successfully. Although I still don't recommend soap, for those of you who can't do without it to wash your face, here are some things you need to know about soap before you wash your face with it again tonight or go shopping for a new one sometime in the future.

What most of us believe is that the tight sensation we feel on the face after washing with soap means the face is clean. You know the feeling I'm talking about—where if you open your mouth it pulls the skin around your eyes? The more squeaky clean your skin feels, the better off you are, right? Wrong! That feeling is irritated, dried-out skin and nothing else. But the difficulty with asking someone to break a soap habit is that soap really does clean the skin thoroughly. Unfortunately, too often it cleans *too* thoroughly, and that can be irritating! After washing with soap, if your skin feels tight for more than two minutes, you will have to run to your moisturizer to prevent the skin from feeling pulled and taut; or, if you have oily skin, the oil will resurface in about ninety seconds no matter how clean you felt initially. If you happen to have combination skin, you will reinforce that dual condition.

The major reason that soap—all soaps—can be a problem is because of the ingredients. Almost always the main ingredients in soap are lard or fats (sodium tallowate, which can clog pores), alkaline cleansing ingredients (sodium cocoate, very drying), or detergent cleansers (also potentially drying). Simply put, lard can make you break out, and alkaline cleansers and some detergent cleansers can be irritating, which may also cause you to break out and to have dry skin.

What about specialty soaps that come in clear bars, have nonsoap-sounding names, or contain creams and emollients that appear to have none of the properties of regular soap? All of the soaps I've looked at—Purpose, Aveeno (oatmeal soaps), Pears, Basis, Neutrogena, and Ivory—all contained sodium tallowate and sodium cocoate. So much for specialty soaps being different. Even worse, the soaps designed for oily or acned skin contained even harsher ingredients. Soaps designed for dry or sensitive skin contained ingredients such as glycerin, petrolatum (mineral oil), or vegetable oil, which might make the face feel somewhat less stiff after you rinse it off, but still won't prevent the irritation the other ingredients create.

Whether or not a bar soap is clear or has a nonsoap-sounding name like "glycerin" or "French milled" does not tell you what it is made of. You can only get that information from the ingredients listing. If you feel some kind of bar soap is your only option, I would strongly suggest trying a few and seeing which ones do not leave your face dry or irritated. You may want to start with Aveeno, Pears, or Neutrogena. But do not use any soaps designed for acned or oily skin. The ingredients in those products are just too harsh.

Here's a rundown of some basic categories of soaps. Remember, just because a product is advertised as being gentle doesn't mean it is.

Castile soaps use olive oil instead of animal fat, but the cleansing agent, sodium hydroxide, is still fairly irritating to the skin.

Transparent soaps look gentle because of their clear appearance, but they often contain harsh cleansing ingredients as well.

Deodorant soaps are always irritating for the face and should only be used on other parts of the body, if at all.

Acne soaps often contain very irritating ingredients in addition to harsh cleansers that, when combined with other acne treatments, can superirritate the skin.

Cosmetic soaps sold at the cosmetics counters for more money than they are worth (the most overpriced being those sold at the Erno Lazlo counters) may be advertised as being gentle or specially formulated, but in this case soap is soap, and they are not any better or differently formulated than the specialty soaps you buy at the drugstore.

Superfatted soaps contain extra oils and fats that supposedly make them more gentle for the face. Basis Soap is one of the most popular superfatted specialty soaps. However gentle, extra glycerin, petrolatum, or beeswax won't prevent irritation. Superfatted soaps may be considered by women with normal skin. They can still be too drying for dry skin and can make oily skin break out.

Oatmeal soaps are supposed to be better at absorbing oil and be less irritating to the skin than other soaps designed for oily skin. I have never found that to be the case, but it may be worth a try for some of you who have oily skin and still want to use soap. Aveeno is the most popular brand on the market, but I would avoid their soap designed for acne. It contains salicylic acid, which can be extremely irritating for anyone.

Natural soaps that contain vitamins, fruits, vegetables, plants, flowers, herbs, aloe, and specialty oils are all gimmicks and serve no purpose on the face. They don't nourish the skin or provide any other health benefits. This is sheer marketing whimsy and nothing more.

I wish I could wholeheartedly recommend one soap over another, but I can't. I still have not found one soap that I think would work better than any other, but if you have found one that you find to be nonirritating, keep on using it and let me know about it.

Summary:

I am not fond of recommending soaps because, for the most part, they are very drying and potentially irritating. But the truth is that many women prefer bar soap. I still prefer Cetaphil Lotion or a similar water-soluble cleanser overall, but perhaps the soap of your choice can be used at night and Cetaphil Lotion can be used in the morning, before applying makeup, to reduce the amount of irritation to the face and to reduce the need for a moisturizer.

Cellular Renewal

Cellular renewal is the nineties term for exfoliating or sloughing the skin, except that in the nineties the cosmetics industry wants you to believe that removing dead skin cells from the surface of the skin will stimulate the growth of new cells. The subject of cellular renewal is a hot topic at the cosmetics counters and in fashion magazines these days. This idea of stimulating cell growth seems to be the latest fad in the endless worldwide pursuit of a way to prevent wrinkles. This is a complicated subject because there is a great deal of benefit to be had in removing dead skin cells from the surface of the skin to make room for other skin cells. But cellular renewal is, as you well may have expected, more fiction than fact.

Cell renewal is a process all skin goes through. After cells are created beneath the surface, they move up through the skin's layers as they change their shape and size, and finally they end up on the surface, where they are ultimately shed. This is the life of a skin cell. The skin we see on the surface, and that several microlayers deeper, is dead. The newly produced skin cells make a trek from this deeper layer of skin to the surface over a period of time. What happens to the skin on this journey from birth to death is what can greatly affect its appearance.

The movement of skin cells from the lower layers of skin to the surface has nothing to do with the way the skin wrinkles. The life and death of skin cells do not affect the collagen and elastin fibers that support the skin. These are not affected by cellular renewal. Collagen and elastin, when exposed to sun over a period of time, deteriorate and this causes wrinkles. So ignore the claim distributors of wrinkle creams make about the creams getting rid of wrinkles because they can supposedly stimulate "cellular renewal."

What can go wrong along the path of these skin cells as they are born, live, die, and are shed? A lot, although not much prior to the age of thirty. Up to that point the skin does a great job of creating new skin cells at an appropriate rate, moving them along upward through the layers of the epidermis in a healthy, smooth manner and then, finally, shedding them when their time is up. But for some of us, particularly as we get older or if we tend to have dry skin, that process is not so smooth, and problems happen along the way that can affect the appearance of skin.

The first potential problem is that skin cell production can slow down, which can leave older, dried-up cells on the surface longer than normal. The second potential problem is that even when skin cell growth is normal, the cells may not shed properly, leaving a buildup on the surface. And the third potential problem is that as the skin cells move through the layers of skin they can become misshapen, stick together unevenly, and have problems retaining water, which can all leave the skin looking dry, dull, and extremely flaky.

Exfoliating the skin, applying good moisturizers, and using nongreasy skin cleansers can alleviate most of these problems. What is a good moisturizer for keeping the cells moving? One that doesn't oversaturate the surface with oils, which can block skin from sloughing off when it's ready, and one that uses ingredients that keep some of the lower layers of skin moist, too (I'll explain more about this in the section on moisturizers). Cleansers must be lightweight and totally rinseable (as I explained earlier), or the greasy film they leave behind can also keep skin from shedding. Exfoliating or sloughing the skin helps the dead surface skin cells shed at a more normal rate to make room for the lower layers of newer skin cells as they finish their trip to the top.

Both dermatologists and cosmetics experts agree (and they rarely agree) that the skin may need help with this process of shedding skin cells and moisturizing the cells on and just beneath the surface. The disagreement exists over whether or not new skin cells can be generated by using cosmetics or pharmaceuticals. Can you generate new skin cells? And if you can, can you generate enough of them to make a difference? Wouldn't you love for me to say there is a way? As I mentioned before, some would say it is as simple as exfoliating the skin—that shedding skin stimulates skin cell production. Others would say that moisturizers can do the job. Unfortunately, there are no studies supporting that concept. I wish there were. But exfoliating the skin is a good step, nevertheless, so read on.

Exfoliating Dry Skin

Exfoliating the skin is a positive skin care step for almost all skin types. The only skin type that may need to shy away from this step altogether is extremely sensitive skin. There is much to be gained from helping the skin shed excess skin cells. But in order to exfoliate the skin, you do need to irritate it. This may sound a bit contradictory; after all, I just spent a long time explaining why being gentle to the skin is important, and now I'm telling you why it is okay to irritate the skin. The fact is, the only way to help exfoliate the skin is by some amount of irritation. The question then becomes, How much irritation is necessary to do the job? My contention is that you can exfoliate the skin in the most gentle way possible and get the best of both worlds.

For exfoliating the skin there are a lot of products out there waiting to peel the money from your pocketbook. Cosmetic scrubs, toners, facial masks, facial peels, abrasive sponges, and facial brushes are all designed to exfoliate. You already know how I feel about toners that contain irritants (which are the only kind that can exfoliate the skin), so there should be no question that this group of products is not to be used for exfoliating. I also mentioned before that I didn't like most facial masks because of their irritating ingredients. Facial peels will be discussed later, in Chapter Four, but suffice it to say that they can be severely irritating for many skin types. Facial brushes are an option, but I find that they are hard to keep clean and can be as irritating as washcloths. Lancôme happens to carry one of the softest facial brushes on the market that I have found, but it is not practical for a wide range of skin types. Abrasive sponges are too irritating and are also very difficult to keep clean. The last group—cosmetics scrubs—is probably the best source for handling the problem of exfoliation.

I know I just said that the most positive way to remove the dead surface layer of skin is by using cosmetic scrubs, but there are also things about these cleansers that I don't like. Many of them contain uneven pieces of cement (silicon), fruit pits, seeds, and other gritty abrasives that can be unnecessarily irritating. The other problem is that these abrasive fragments are not of a uniform shape and can literally cut the skin. Cosmetic scrubs often contain thick waxes and creams mixed with the abrasive substance so you can smooth it more easily over your skin. Waxes can clog pores and leave a film over the face. Some scrub products also contain additional harsh ingredients that are unnecessary and harmful. The last problem with all scrubs—even the one I recommend, which I will get to in just a moment—is that you can easily end up scrubbing off more than is healthful for the skin. You still need to exfoliate, but how to do that gently is the question.

The answer is that the best way to gently exfoliate dry, normal, or sensitive skin is with baking soda mixed with Cetaphil Lotion or with the water-soluble cleanser you are currently using. Why baking soda? Because baking soda is a small-grained salt product that can work as an effective scrub on your face. There is nothing else mixed in with it, so you don't have to worry about other harsh ingredients or wax thickeners that can irritate the skin, clog pores, or not rinse off thoroughly. I find this to be the simplest yet most effective solution to the problem of exfoliating dry skin gently.

Baking soda is really much better than the scrubs you buy in the drugstore or at the cosmetics counters. Baking soda is an anti-inflammatory agent—it can reduce redness, irritation, and itching. For example, if you got a bee sting, you wouldn't put honey and almond pits or a buffing puff on it, but you might use a poultice of baking soda to reduce the swelling. Finally, baking soda is not a grit suspended in a cosmetic base. Cosmetic scrubs often contain preservatives, coloring agents, and fragrances that can irritate the skin and waxes that can clog the pores. For the money (89 cents for a medium-size box), you can't find a product on the market that works any more effectively to exfoliate the skin.

Summary:

When you have dry skin, too many dried-up cells are trying to jump ship and there are not enough water-filled ones to take their place. This crowd of cells, each waiting its turn, creates a backup of flaky, dull-looking skin. If you then put a moisturizer only on top of those skin cells to reduce the flakiness, the dried-up skin cells ready to be shed are held up under the oil/wax layer of the cream. To make matters worse, the more dead skin builds up and is unable to shed, the less effective is the moisturizer. The dried-up skin cells can actually block the moisturizer from reaching the water-filled cells in the layers below, which may lose their water while they wait too long for their turn to get to the surface. Scrub-type cleansers that help slough the skin can prevent this backup from taking place. The question isn't whether or not the skin needs help with this exfoliating process, because it does; the question is, How much help does it need and how can you do it gently?

Directions: *After you have removed all your makeup and rinsed off your cleanser, squeeze about two tablespoons of Cetaphil Lotion into the palm of your hand and then pour about one or two tablespoons of baking soda over it. Mix the two together in the palms of your hands and massage over the face. Be gentle and do not overscrub. Rinse thoroughly. Do not leave any traces of the mixture behind on the face. For most dry or mature skin types, this process can be repeated two or three times a week. How often needs to be judged by you. The main things to watch out for are irritation and tenderness. If you notice any irritation, cut down the frequency or reduce the amount of time you massage the skin.*

Note: *Always keep two things in mind when using baking soda. You can overdo the baking soda, so do not overscrub. Judge how often to use the baking soda by paying attention to your skin. If your skin is dry and feeling very sensitive, be ever so careful with your application, and perhaps do this step only once or twice a week.*

Exfoliating Oily Skin

One of the reasons a pore can get clogged with oil is that surface skin cells that should be falling off the skin instead fall into the pore and get stuck. The more skin cells that build up in the pore, the more oil can be prevented from flowing easily out of the pore, and the result can be a blemish. The skin cells that should be shedding on a regular, daily basis are being held back. One of the things that is keeping the cells from sloughing off is the very oil (sebum) your skin produces. Oil is a sticky substance that spreads over the skin, settling mostly where the active oil glands are, in the center of the face. The oil works as an adhesive, keeping the shedding skin from going where it is supposed to go—off the face and onto the floor. The repetition of this occurring every day—dead skin cells building up in the pore—is why skin problems can show up. The skin cells pile up inside the pore, getting trapped by the stickiness of the oil, which blocks the oil flow to the surface and clogs the pore.

One of the ways to keep pores from getting clogged is to help the skin cells shed as freely as possible so they don't get trapped inside the pore. Exfoliating oily as well as acned skin is very beneficial. The more you keep the skin moving off the face, the less cell debris can fill the pore. The same process that works for dry skin works equally well for oily skin. The only difference is that it needs to be done more often. The oil on the surface of the skin needs to be eliminated when you clean your face, and then the same scrub—baking soda—can be used to remove excess skin cells. The benefits can be amazing when you use a gentle scrub on oily skin that tends to break out.

Directions: *After the face is cleansed with a water-soluble cleanser (I prefer Cetaphil Lotion, but those with severely oily skin may prefer one of the others I mentioned in the cleanser/soap section), pour two table-spoons of baking soda directly into the palm of your hand. Add a drop or two of water, turning the baking soda into a slight paste, and then massage this mixture directly over the face, putting a bit extra on blemishes. Depending on your skin type and how much your skin can handle, this step can be repeated every night or twice a day. For those of you with more sensitive or mature oily skin, you may mix the Cetaphil Lotion with the baking soda and use that as your scrub. Or you can still use the baking soda directly, but perhaps only three times a week instead of every day. It is up to you, and you alone, to gauge the frequency of using the baking soda on the face. For those with very sensitive skin or those with spot breakouts, you can massage the baking soda only on the blemish itself and nowhere else and then rinse well.*

Note: *There are other factors besides skin cells blocking a pore that can cause blemishes, but this theory about skin cells getting stuck inside a pore and clogging it is a basic one. I will explain more in Chapter Five on acne.*

What Do Toners Tone?

It is my fervent opinion that all toners, no matter what they are called—astringents, fresheners, pore cleansers, or clarifying lotions, Sea Breeze or witch hazel or a toner made by Borghese or Estée Lauder—as long as they contain irritating ingredients, are bad for the skin. They are bad for all skin, even oily and acned skin types. The only toners, astringents, clarifying lotions, fresheners, and pore cleansers you should ever consider using are those that are 100 percent irritant free.

The primary ingredient in most toners—even many of those designed for dry skin—is usually SD alcohol with a number following it. That's ethanol alcohol—the kind used to sterilize medical instruments, the kind you would never put on a cut or wound, and the kind that is a known irritant. If you thought that astringents or toners that contain alcohol provided a good disinfectant for the skin, you're wrong. In order for an astringent containing alcohol to be an effective disinfectant, it needs to contain 60 to 70 percent pure alcohol. When you purchase most astringents you're primarily getting watered-down alcohol in the 20 to 40 percent range. At even a 40 percent level, you're not getting an effective disinfectant, although you are getting an effective irritant.

> Let me set the record straight. Astringents do not close pores; they do not deep-clean pores; and they do not reduce oil production.

There are other irritating ingredients to be found in toner-type products: acetone, citrus (lemon, grapefruit, and orange juice are incredibly irritating to the skin because of their high acid content), salicylic acid, camphor, mint, peppermint, menthol, boric acid, and witch hazel. Alcohol should be avoided as well as all these other ingredients.

The funny thing—well, maybe not so funny—is that, regardless of the price category, all toners are pretty much the same. The ingredients are astoundingly similar. Water and alcohol, some coloring agents, a little glycerin, and maybe some allantoin is not what I would call exotic. But regardless of the price tag, alcohol burns the skin, and that is never beneficial.

What do toners, astringents, and the rest of them do? When they contain irritants, all they do is irritate the skin. Actually, it is easier to say what these toners and astringents don't do. Let me set the record straight. Astringents do not close pores; they do not deep-clean pores; and they do not reduce oil production. All irritation does to a pore is to temporarily swell it, which can make the pore look smaller for maybe a few minutes. Toners that contain alcohol can remove the surface oil from the skin, but if you've cleansed the skin properly, there should be no surface oil left. You can't get inside a pore with a toner to deep-clean it; if you could, we would all have spotless, empty pores. Most of all, toners do not reduce oil production. Quite the contrary: because irritating ingredients can severely irritate the nerve endings and because the nerve endings are attached to the oil glands, they can stimulate oil production, which can make pores larger. It is a vicious cycle. Astringents and toners worsen the very problem they are supposedly designed to handle.

In essence, stay away from all cosmetics that contain alcohol and other irritating ingredients. When it comes to alcohol, do not be confused by cosmetics that contain ingredients that sound like alcohol but are not. For example, cetyl alcohol or alcohol esters are not the type of alcohol I'm warning you about. Remember, the ingredients label will list the alcohol as "SD alcohol" followed by a number. That's the kind to avoid.

You may be wondering about the toners, astringents, fresheners, pore cleansers, and clarifying lotions that claim to be made especially for sensitive skin or dry skin or are labeled "gentle" or "hypoallergenic." More times than I care to count, I have found that these very products contain an extremely irritating assortment of ingredients and would be the last thing I would recommend for sensitive or allergy-prone skin. Then there are the times where the salespeople have promised me that the toners they are selling don't contain that much alcohol. That is misleading. If you are looking for a gentle toner, diluted alcohol is still alcohol, and even watered down it can be irritating to the skin. Alcohol isn't always the irritating ingredient; if any of the other ingredients I've mentioned above are present, watered down or not, they can be irritating as well.

So what about these new irritant-free toners on the market? They are a fine alternative for that extra cleansing step after removing the cleanser. They won't close pores and they won't deep-clean, but they will leave a cool, smooth feeling on the face, remove any last traces of makeup or oil, and soothe the skin. That makes irritant-free toners a wonderful cleansing aid. What is in these products that make them beneficial to the skin? They usually are a plain concoction of water, glycerin, and allantoin, accompanied by a fancy price.

Summary:

There are no toners available that can close pores. Toners that contain irritants can damage the skin. Irritant-free toners, however, can be a soothing, refreshing extra step to clean the last remnants of oil and makeup off the face.

Directions: *After your cleanser has been rinsed off and your face has been dried, soak a piece of cotton with the toner and go over your entire face without pulling the skin. You may want to repeat this step a second time if you notice any traces of makeup on the cotton. Because the toner you are using now is irritant free, there should be no cause for redness or inflammation unless you are allergic to the product.*

How to Survive Oily Skin at Any Age

Oily skin is definitely a problem, and too much oily skin is annoying. Regardless of how little or how much, it always feels like *too* much. Oily-skin paranoia is hard to talk anyone out of. Fighting the battle of a constant oil slick on the face is no fun. And for most of us, along with the constant oil flow there is the almost constant struggle against breakouts. From this side of the world, dry skin would be a blessing. I'm not going to preach that you have to love your oily skin, but neither am I going to encourage you to hate it. Hating oily skin doesn't help. The more we hate it, the more we do things that abuse the face. Somewhere there is a middle ground where you can learn to stop trying to sear the oils off your skin and come to terms with a more gentle approach, which in the long run will be better for your skin.

This one is hard to believe, but oil on the face is really good stuff. Oil is needed to create a barrier between your skin and the environment. The oil film prevents the air from absorbing the moisture from the surface of the skin, which keeps the skin moist. Those of us who have active oil glands rarely have to use moisturizers because we were born with our own moisturizer built in. Why some of us have more oil than others seems to be related primarily to genetics—you inherited your oily skin trait from your parents.

The oiliest areas on the face are the nose, chin, cheeks, and the center of the forehead because that is where the most oil glands are located. That comes with being human. There are fewer active oil glands on the sides of the face. No wonder many of us tend to have combination skin—it's the way the system works.

This is a good time to clarify what exactly this oil is that causes so much grief on the skin. First of all, the word *oil* is very misleading. From surface appearance we assume that the oil inside the pore is similar to mineral oil or olive oil. That just isn't the case. The oil underneath our skin, in the pore itself, is hard. It is the same kind of waxy substance produced in our ears. This oil/wax pushes its way to the surface, liquefying at surface temperature.

> Being gentle to your face won't eliminate your oily skin, but using all those irritating products designed for oily skin never got rid of the oil either.

Once we understand that the oil we see on the surface of the skin was originally a semihard, whitish, waxlike substance secreted by our oil glands, we can better comprehend why excess oil production can wreak so much havoc on the skin. It isn't liquid oil that gets backed up inside the pore, it is a semihard waxy material that is capable of stretching a pore and creating solid bumps. The question is, How do you keep this oil/wax flow from backing up?

The popular assumption that oil can be dried up, which has been around for decades, explains why there are so many alcohol-based products on the market for oily-skin problems. The supposition is that since alcohol effectively degreases the surface of the skin, it must be effective for ridding the skin of oil. And to some extent that is true. However, the folly in this logic is that applying alcohol to the skin only removes the surface oil (which should have already been removed when you washed the face). Alcohol cannot reach the wax inside the pore. The other problem is that the irritation imparted on the skin by using alcohol (or any other irritant) makes the oil gland produce *more* oil because the irritation stimulates the nerves, which activate the oil gland, thereby creating more oil. How many times have you applied an alcohol-based toner to your face only to find that 90 seconds later the oil resurfaced? You haven't changed the oil situation—but you've severely irritated the skin.

One of the two ways to survive oily skin is to realize that you don't have to beat up the face to get rid of oil, and the other is to calm down oil production by treating your skin gently and calming down the nerve endings first. Being gentle to your face won't eliminate your oily skin, but using all those irritating products designed for oily skin never got rid of the oil either. In fact, those products made the skin more oily and, in addition to the problem of oil, the irritating ingredients caused the skin to become inflamed, red, swollen, and dry. Instead of having one skin type—oily skin—you've ended up with three. There isn't a magic cure for oily skin, but you can live with it peacefully and keep the surface of the skin looking smoother by reducing the skin problems that accompany irritation. The next two steps will give you some helpful tools that are staples in my skin care routine for oily and acned skin types.

Reminder: *A major way to avoid complicating or worsening oily skin is eliminate using a moisturizer of any kind—oil free or otherwise. I'll explain more about this later, but for now just understand that oily skin is not necessarily in need of extra moisture if you don't do anything to dry it out.*

A Special Toner for Blemishes

Oily or acned skin can benefit from the use of alcohol-free, nonirritating toners just as the other skin types can. But for oily skin that has blemishes and blackheads, that won't be enough. What I recommend as a toner strictly for these skin problems is three percent hydrogen peroxide solution, which you can buy in the drugstore, grocery store or convenience store for about 69 cents bottle.

Although your initial reaction might be to think that three percent hydrogen peroxide solution sounds like it is too strong for the skin to handle, nothing could be further from the truth. Unlike an alcohol-based toner or astringent, a three percent solution of hydrogen peroxide is an extremely efficient and gentle disinfectant. A three percent hydrogen peroxide solution can easily be used in place of any astringent, toner, or freshener, and it will do far more for the skin without irritating it.

Hydrogen peroxide is an effective disinfectant at a three percent solution level—three percent hydrogen peroxide to 97 percent water—whereas alcohol, in order to be an effective disinfectant, needs to be at a 70 percent solution level. That makes alcohol useful only at a very toxic concentration. A three percent hydrogen peroxide solution isn't toxic at all. It is gentle enough to be recommended by dentists as a mouthwash to help prevent gum disease. You could never do that with an astringent.

A three percent hydrogen peroxide solution does not burn or react on the skin unless the skin is abraded. Where the skin is open, the peroxide will fizz and turn white. Alcohol does just the opposite—it burns the skin upon exposure no matter what comes in contact with it. A three percent hydrogen peroxide solution, with continual use, can change the color of blackheads by turning them back to white. (It does this by bleaching out the color of the melanin cells that have fallen into the pore, which turned the pore dark in the first place.) Alcohol just sits there on the surface of the skin and torments the nerve endings.

By now you may be wondering why the strongest alcohol-based astringents and toners in every skin care line are designed for oily skin. I've wondered the same thing myself. Lord knows I've tried enough of them in the past, and one after the other they all did the same thing—irritated my skin. My only excuse for this repeated abuse of my face is that those were the days when I thought irritation was making my skin better, even though it visibly looked worse. I kept hoping that would change, and it did, but not because of astringents. My skin didn't have a chance back then. It changed when I started treating my skin gently.

Another question you may also be asking is, "If the three percent hydrogen peroxide solution is so wonderful, why don't the cosmetics companies use it in their products?" That's a very good question. The answer lies in the problem of product stability. Chemicals must remain stable and interact favorably with each other to make a cosmetic formula work. A three percent hydrogen peroxide solution is a highly unstable ingredient. It can decompose upon contact with sunlight and air. That's why three percent hydrogen peroxide solution comes packaged in those little brown bottles and should be purchased in small quantities—it can break down very easily and become plain everyday water. On the other hand, alcohol is chosen for its ability to be mixed with practically anything and remain intact for long periods of time. Alcohol also degreases the skin, but I've already explained that severe degreasing can hurt the skin.

After painting such a rosy picture of three percent hydrogen peroxide solution, there are, as you well may have expected, two side effects you should know about before you start to use it. Be careful with it around your hairline and eyebrows, since hair will turn blond when soaked repeatedly with peroxide. While you may appreciate some inexpensive highlighting along your hairline, it definitely isn't for everyone. Protecting your eyebrows may be more of a nuisance at first, but you'll get the hang of it. The second caution is that three percent hydrogen peroxide solution can be drying for those with ultrasensitive skin or very dry skin. But the only reason those skin types should be using the three percent hydrogen peroxide solution anyway is if they have a problem with blackheads or breakouts. If not, there is no reason to use the peroxide.

Summary:

A three percent hydrogen peroxide solution is a good disinfectant to use over blemishes. It changes the color of blackheads from black to white, causes minimal to no irritation to the skin, and is even less expensive than baking soda.

Directions: *Use the three percent hydrogen peroxide solution as you would any other toner, but be careful to avoid the hairline and eyebrows. Only those with blemishes and blackheads should be following this step, and using the three percent hydrogen peroxide solution in only those areas. If your skin is dry or very sensitive and has breakouts, use the three percent peroxide sparingly and only over those problem areas. You can also dampen the cotton ball with a little water before soaking it with the three percent hydrogen peroxide solution. The extra dilution should help cut almost any risk of irritation.*

A Unique Facial Mask for Blemishes

The second tool in your survival kit for blemishes and oily skin is milk of magnesia as a facial mask. (Aren't you glad I didn't mean for you to take it internally?) What could be in milk of magnesia that would make it suitable as a facial mask? Why not good old-fashioned mud masks that are available from many cosmetics lines? All milk of magnesia is, is liquid magnesium. What is liquid magnesium? It's a simple combination of magnesium powder and water. When those two ingredients are mixed together they become magnesium hydroxide, or milk of magnesia. Besides what it is traditionally used for, milk of magnesia has two properties that make it excellent topically for oily skin and acned skin. It can absorb a lot of oil, and it is a very effective disinfectant—exactly what you need when dealing with oily skin and blemishes.

The problem with traditional mud masks is that they are not as effective as milk of magnesia. Mud masks contain clay, which like magnesium is an earth mineral but cannot absorb oil as well as magnesium can. Mud masks often contain other irritating ingredients that can make the skin look red and inflamed. Milk of magnesia is not an irritant and contains no other ingredients that can hurt the skin. For the money, it would be worth it to find out if I'm right.

Directions: *After you've finished washing your face with the water-soluble cleanser and the baking soda, or whether or not you use the baking soda, and after you use the three percent hydrogen peroxide solution and let it dry, you can then apply the milk of magnesia in a layer generously over the face. Apply the milk of magnesia with your fingers or a cotton ball. It tends to be a little runny, so be patient as you build up an opaque layer over the face. Leave this on until it dries, which should take no longer than ten to fifteen minutes, then rinse well. Milk of magnesia is difficult to rinse off, so be sure to rinse thoroughly. Regardless of skin type, never leave the milk of magnesia on overnight.*

Caution: *The three percent hydrogen peroxide solution and milk of magnesia are only to be used if you have a problem with blemishes and/or oily skin. If not, it is not necessary for you to include these items in your skin care routine.*

Moisturizers—The Good News and the Bad

Moisturizers are frustrating—not because they're complicated, but because they aren't. More to the point, the cosmetics industry continues to portray moisturizers as bottled scientific miracles, and they aren't. I need to penetrate a lot of fantasy and provocative rhetoric in order to explain the truth about what moisturizers can and can't do. One thing is certain: the truth isn't nearly as profound and alluring as the stuff you will read in the fashion magazines or hear at the cosmetics counters. For starters, I'm not going to illustrate my information with glossy pictures of perfect-skinned half-naked teenagers. Nevertheless, I will present it to you the best way I know how and hope that by now you are willing to be less seduced by fancy packaging and vague advertising language.

When it comes to moisturizers, there is good news and bad news. The good news is that there are some remarkably effective moisturizers on the market in all price ranges that can take care of dry skin beautifully. There are also wonderful sunscreens of SPF 15 or greater available at all prices that can prevent wrinkling by keeping the sun off the face. The bad news is that most moisturizers do not contain a sunscreen of SPF 15 or greater, and they cannot do a thing about preventing or changing wrinkles. Remember, it is the sun that causes wrinkles, not dry skin.

The Truth About Wrinkle Creams

Most women, of all ages, are concerned about moisturizing their skin. Twenty-year-old women, regardless of skin type, will say "moisturizers" when asked what skin care products they think are most important. There are thousands of moisturizers, and they all claim to be able to reduce the appearance of wrinkles. We spend a lot of money trying to find the best one—the one with the most scientific-sounding promises or the one with the latest ingredients or the one that someone told us could deliver youthful, moist skin. Yet our search isn't getting us anywhere. Why are so many of us willing to spend our money on little more than a lot of hype and promotion? As you may already suspect, the reasons are rooted in our fears of growing up.

> The emotions get involved because our egos get hooked into wanting the impossible.

Moisturizing the skin is one of the most emotion-packed, sensitive areas I can think of in skin care. The emotions get involved because our egos get hooked into wanting the impossible. Wrinkling is a hard-core visual sign of mortality and waning youth. Many women want to believe that if they use a moisturizer—a *good* moisturizer—they can prevent or at least slow down the inevitable process of wrinkling. I would like to believe that, too, but it's not the truth.

Unlike other skin care problems, the issue of wrinkles has an impact on almost everybody regardless of race, religion, sex, or ethnic background. That's because at some point everyone who has spent any time in the sun without a sunscreen is going to wrinkle sooner than they would have if they had stayed out of the sun. There is no other skin condition that is quite so permanent (face-lifts notwithstanding) and quite so inevitable (it's hard to avoid the sun). Wrinkles will never just get up and go away by themselves, so don't get sucked into buying wrinkle creams.

The primary reason that the subject of moisturizers is so convoluted and misunderstood is the misinformation that accompanies this overly advertised group of products. The cosmetics industry wants you to believe that moisturizers alleviate or prevent wrinkling by reducing dry skin, keeping the environment off the face, and stimulating cellular renewal. None of that is true. Moisturizers have *no* permanent or long-lasting effect on wrinkles.

> Dry skin and wrinkling are not associated; they have nothing to do with each other. If we could understand this basic truth about our skin, we would stop slathering expensive creams on our faces in the hope of preventing wrinkles.

The really big myth that lives on and on is that dry skin causes wrinkles. The cosmetics industry has spent a lot of money convincing us that dry skin and wrinkling are associated. To put it simply, dry skin and wrinkling are not associated; they have nothing to do with each other. If we could understand this basic truth about our skin, we would stop slathering expensive creams on our faces in the hope of preventing wrinkles. I know that's hard to believe, because from a superficial perspective, dry skin looks (I repeat, *looks*) more wrinkled than moist skin. But the similarities and associations start and stop there. These are the facts: dry skin is caused by the inability of the surface layers of skin to retain water, or dehydration. When dehydrated skin "looks" wrinkled, it is quickly corrected by placing a moisturizer over it. Permanent wrinkles, the ones caused by the deterioration of the collagen and elastin in the dermis due to sun exposure, are not affected by moisturizers of any kind.

Consider this: if dry skin caused wrinkling, teenagers with dry skin would wrinkle, but they don't. Also, if dry skin caused wrinkles, women with oily skin would never wrinkle, and as I can personally and professionally attest, we do.

There probably aren't many women out there who have any idea of what they're buying when it comes to a moisturizer. Yet, they believe or trust it will impede or reverse the wrinkling process. Even those who know the truth about what moisturizers can actually do often continue to buy wrinkle creams anyway, just in case they might be wrong and the cosmetics industry right.

What the Sun Does to the Face

Repeated exposure to the sun affects the skin in the following ways: it destroys the collagen and elastin support tissues in the dermis (the deepest layers of living skin); it radically thins the lower layers of the epidermis (the dead layer of protective surface skin); it thickens the very surface of the skin we see, causing brown or ashen skin spots; it causes the skin to look yellow or ashen; it destroys the skin's blood vessels by destroying the collagen and elastin that support the blood vessels; it destroys the skin's immune tissue; and most important, the sun causes 95 percent of all skin cancers (there are over 500,000 newly diagnosed cases of basal cell carcinomas each year and over 7,000 deaths). The other thing the sun can do to the skin is create skin discolorations. This is a problem for women of all colors. Sun-damaged skin can become freckled or spotted. These sun spots are usually uneven in appearance and can grow. The skin can also get patches of rough-textured thickened skin. These areas on the skin are possibly a pre-cancerous condition and should be checked out by a competent dermatologist. Again, none of this has anything to do with age, only with repeated sun exposure. But the most shocking news of all, is that most of this damage occurs before one reaches thirty. Clearly, when it comes to the sun's impact on the skin, we're not talking about wrinkles alone.

Genetic Aging Versus Photoaging—An Update

Genetic aging refers to the natural process of the human system slowing down, stopping, or degenerating as it ages. Photoaging refers to what happens to an individual's skin with repeated exposure to the sun. Recent studies over the past ten years, most conducted by Dr. Albert Kligman, the inventor of Retin-A, seem to support the notion that we are *not* genetically preprogrammed to wrinkle. Although many youthful support systems do break down as we get older, skin, in terms of wrinkling, isn't one of them! Wrinkling we can prevent, sagging we cannot. But we can't prevent wrinkling with wrinkle creams. The only way to prevent wrinkling is to keep the sun totally off the face. It is that simple.

> Repeated sun exposure thins the lower layers of skin and thickens the outer layers of skin.

Photoaged skin differs in both structure and texture from skin that has not been exposed to the sun. Remember, sun-damaged skin is not necessarily indicated by the sagging skin around the jowls or eyelids. Photoaged skin is most apparent on the cheeks, around the eyes, chest, backs of the hands, and, if you've had short hair most of your life, the back of the neck. In actuality, sun-damaged skin can occur wherever the skin has been exposed on a regular basis to the sun. Sunbathers are not the only ones subject to the effects of the sun, although they are more likely to show damage sooner and more severely. The sun can damage our skin when we walk outside and drive to the office as well as when we sunbathe.

Still not convinced that the sun is what wrinkles the face and nothing else? Take the following intimate test I call "The Backside Test of Photoaging."

This test is most startling to women who have some amount of wrinkling present on the face. If you don't have any wrinkles yet, you can give this test anonymously to any woman who has sun-damaged skin the next time you're at your local health club. Simply adapt the rules as you go.

Here's what to do. Next time you find yourself completely naked and in proximity to a full-length mirror, stand in front of it and examine the skin's appearance on your face, hands, neck, and chest. Then examine the skin on your buttocks. Note the differences. You should try to be as objective as possible, putting all personal feelings on the back burner. The test is most revealing when you take note of exactly the way the skin looks in terms of tone, color, elasticity, and texture.

What you will notice is that the skin on the buttocks is fairly even in color with minimal to no signs of skin discoloration. The areas that have been exposed to the sun all your life will be more yellow (for Caucasian and Asian skin) or ashy (for African-American skin colors). Even if there are surface capillaries visible, the skin will be an overall dull, sallow shade. The skin's texture will be crisscrossed with lines, and the eyes and forehead may have deep furrows.

After assessing all this you will have noticed that the major difference between the skin that has been exposed to the sun and the skin that hasn't is the absence of wrinkles. The backside, in comparison to the face, is smooth and even-colored whereas the skin on the face and hands is not. Smooth, wrinkle-free skin is only possible when it has not been exposed to the sun.

To take it a step further, Dr. Kligman has done studies that compare the skin of eighty-year-old Japanese Buddhist monks to eighty-year-old Native Americans. What his research reveals is that the Japanese monks, who have a totally monastic existence most of the lives and rarely venture outside, have no wrinkles anywhere on the face. That is in direct contrast to Native Americans, who spend a great deal of time outdoors and as a result have very leathery, wrinkled facial skin.

Now that you understand what causes wrinkles, you can start worrying less about which wrinkle cream to use and start focusing on wearing a sunscreen of SPF 15 or greater. It won't change the damage that has already occurred, but it can prevent further damage from happening.

There is no such thing as a safe tan.

Become addicted to using a sunscreen. Sunlight on bare, unprotected flesh prematurely destroys the supportive skin fibers. Therefore, during the day, sunscreen is more important than a moisturizer. All the moisturizers in the world cannot undo what the sun, over time, can do to the face.

Suntan lotion ads would have you believe that as long as you use a sunscreen you can tan safely. Or you may have heard deceptive information about how tanning slowly is a way to prevent wrinkles or skin cancer. If tanning safely means not getting a sunburn, you indeed can do that by using a sunscreen, but that won't prevent wrinkles or skin cancer. You can tan slowly and take a longer time to turn brown, but that also won't prevent wrinkling or skin cancer. A very practical, although grossly dull, idea is to avoid exposing your skin, especially your face, to direct sunlight altogether. But who wants to avoid sunlight? No one. The answer is sunscreen with an SPF of 15 or greater, which can keep the sun totally off the face and therefore prevent wrinkles and skin cancer.

What do you need to know in order to buy and use an effective sunscreen? There are only a handful of guidelines necessary to make this part of skin care second nature.

1 The all-important SPF number is something most of us already understand; what we might be confused about is what number to use. In order to keep the damaging effects of the rays entirely off the face, every dermatologist I've interviewed recommends using a sunscreen of SPF 15 or greater. Anything less than that and you will leave your skin vulnerable to the sun.

2 Wear a sunscreen under your makeup every day to fight the daily effects of sun exposure. Even if you are only outside for a brief time, over the years, 365 days a year, that small exposure to the sun can culminate in sun-damaged skin. If you have dry skin, look for a sunscreen that contains the same ingredients you would find in your moisturizer and wear it under your makeup. It is not necessary to wear a sunscreen and moisturizer at the same time.

3 Foundations that contain sunscreen are a good idea, but as of this writing I've yet to find one that contains a sunscreen with

an SPF of 15. Most foundations that contain a sunscreen have one with an SPF of 8 or less. That is not really enough, but it is better than nothing. If you are wearing a moisturizer that contains a sunscreen of SPF 15, it doesn't hurt to wear a foundation that also has a sunscreen in it. The extra protection is just that much better for the skin. If you do find a foundation that has a sunscreen of SPF 15 (and it matches your skin color), that is all you need during the day to protect the skin.

4 Many people are allergic to the active ingredients in sunscreens. PABA is a popular sunscreen ingredient, but it can cause allergic reactions. Thankfully, PABA is not the only sunscreen ingredient on the market. There are dozens of different ingredients that are currently being used in sunscreens, and it is unlikely you would be allergic to all of them. Keep up the search until you find one that works. If after trying several brands you are still having problems finding one you are not allergic to, it is best that you discuss this with your dermatologist.

5 There are no differences in the effectiveness of an expensive sunscreen with an SPF of 15 and an inexpensive sunscreen with an SPF of 15. Nivea, Mary Kay, Johnson & Johnson, Coppertone, and many other brands that you can find at the drugstore make excellent sunscreens, and you can even wear them under your makeup.

6 If you are going to be spending time in the sun, you must apply your sunscreen liberally—a lot is better than a little to assure an even, complete application. One of the reasons I recommend inexpensive sunscreens is because you are less likely to be liberal with a $35 sunscreen than you are with a $7 sunscreen, and there is absolutely no difference in their effectiveness.

7 If you plan on wearing a hat or spending your time in the shade and you think that will be enough to protect you from the sun, think again. Sand, snow, water, and even concrete can reflect the sun's rays from the ground directly onto your face and damage the skin.

8 Clouds and haze pose harmful problems for the skin when it comes to sun exposure. We tend to think that if we can't see the sun it can't affect us, but the opposite is true. Clouds, haze, and smog filter out some of the sun's rays—but not the ultraviolet, burning ones.

9 When sunbathing, do not forget to apply sunscreen to your ears, lips, underarms, feet, and balding scalps—these are all subject to sun exposure and are often passed over as we diligently apply sunscreen to other parts of the body.

10 Sunscreens do not correct past sun-damaged skin, and sun damage began the first time you were wheeled outside as an infant. From a very young age, everyone should wear a sunscreen. Infants, children, and teenagers can prevent future problems by starting now.

11 Sunscreens do not last all day and need to be reapplied, particularly if you are going to be swimming or exercising. Be sure to reapply your sunscreen immediately after these activities. There are waterproof sunscreens that do not wash off immediately when you get wet, but it is still recommended that you reapply them every two hours.

12 Certain medications, including birth-control pills, tranquilizers, antibiotics, antidepressants, and Retin-A are possibly phototoxic, which means they can be dangerous to use in conjunction with prolonged sun exposure, even if you do apply a sunscreen. Check with your physician before using any prescription drug and spending time in the sun.

13 Skin cancer in the beginning stages may show up as either a slight skin discoloration, an irregularly shaped or discolored mole, or a persistent deep, enlarged blackhead around the eye, cheek, or neck. If you notice anything that you suspect may be a problem, ask your doctor immediately. It may save your face or life!

14 The sunnier the climate, the greater your chances of skin cancer. Also, in areas such as Australia, Fiji, Tahiti, and New Zealand, where ozone depletion is taking place, skin cancer is increasing at an alarming rate. Sunscreen in these areas is not an option; it is mandatory.

If you participate in outdoor sports such as running or skiing, be sure to carry a tube of Chapstick or clear lipstick that contains an SPF of 15 or greater. This is a convenient, easy way to glide protection over the face frequently any time you need it. Chapstick and clear lipstick protect the face from the wind as well as the sun.

What if wearing a sunscreen makes you break out in blemishes? I have personally struggled with this problem for a long time and I wish I had a great, immediate solution, but I don't. All moisturizers of any kind make me break out. Whether they claim to be oil free, hypoallergenic, designed for oily skin, pure and natural, or come in the gel form, I always break out. Finding a sunscreen that won't make me break out has been impossible. When I'm out in the sun for long periods of time, I put up with the resulting bumps and wear a sunscreen anyway because I'm willing to suffer a few blemishes in order to protect my skin from the sun. A few blemishes cannot be compared to skin cancer and severe wrinkling. During a regular working day, what I have chosen to do is wear a foundation that contains an SPF of 8. It isn't as good as wearing sunscreen with an SPF of 15, but it is better than nothing and my foundation doesn't make me break out as creams and gels do. But, as soon as they start making foundations with an SPF of 15 I will be the first one to to give them a try.

Alert: *Tanning machines offer no protection from the sun, regardless of the claims made about the "special" ultraviolet radiation these machines supposedly emit. The truth is that all tanning is bad for the skin.*

Understanding the SPF Number

The SPF number you should use is based on "burn time." If it takes your nontanned skin twenty minutes in the sun to burn, you multiply that time by the SPF number and that is how long you can stay in the sun without burning if you use that sunscreen: 20 minutes × SPF 6 equals 120 minutes of sun exposure without burning. Or if it takes your skin ten minutes in the sun to burn and you are thinking of using a sunscreen with an SPF of 8, the calculation would look like this: 10 minutes × SPF 8 equals 80 minutes of protection from the sun before you would burn. When it comes to the sun, the greater the protection, the less chance you will have to worry about premature aging and cancer.

What to Do After the Sun

This question is a bit loaded because it assumes you have been sitting in the sun, which I absolutely do not want you to do. I actually feel a bit hypocritical relaying information about "after-sun" products, but those of you who unwisely indulge in tanning should not get ripped off by wasting your money on after-sun products. What are after-sun products? They are the creams and lotions that mistakenly offer the hope of helping you keep your tan for as long as possible. So-called after-sun creams and lotions are nothing more than moisturizers. There is absolutely nothing special or unique in these products. If you are operating under the assumption that slathering on moisturizers will somehow keep the skin from peeling and keep your tan around longer, think again. When skin cells need to come off, they need to come off, and trying to prevent that from happening can make the skin look dull and flaky. It is similar to what happens to dry skin when too many dead skin cells are left on the surface of the face. The skin can look drier than it is. Using your regular moisturizer on a tan is fine; using an after-sun product is unnecessary, and overmoisturizing can be a problem.

Tanning Without Damaging the Skin

I wish I could tell you that there is a convincing way to create a fake tan, but there isn't. There are no products available that create a realistic, problem-free Hawaiian tan. A fake tan that looks fake is not attractive. I have never, ever been an advocate of using bronzing gels, bronzing powders, or darker shades of foundations to add color to the face. Any time you try to change the color of your face to a darker shade you inevitably end up with an obvious line of demarcation at the jawline. Your face will have a mask of brown instead of the "natural" tan look you were hoping for. If you think you can avoid this masked look by blending the color down onto the neck, forget it—you can't. You'll only substitute one problem for another—namely makeup on your collar, which is not a good idea. And the rest of your body will still look noticeably lighter. The cosmetics salespeople may tell you their bronzers deliver a "sheer" golden brown glow to the face, but any shade that is different from your own skin color, no matter how sheer, will look different from the rest of you.

A fake tan that looks fake is not attractive.

Along with bronzing powders and gels, self-tanning creams are also being sold at cosmetics counters for the purpose of creating a sunless tan. These products are supposed to impart a convincing, semipermanent, golden brown color to the skin, and to some extent, that is exactly what they do. Unfortunately, how real the tan looks is a matter of opinion, and using the products can create problems that are difficult, if not impossible, to avoid.

Self-tanning creams contain an ingredient called dihydroxyacetone. By itself, dihydroxyacetone looks like a white powder. Skin may become a light shade of golden brown a few hours after you've applied the cream. You can control how dark a tan you build by controlling the frequency of application. The effect is semipermanent and does not rub off on clothes. It is considered safe to use all over your body, if you are not allergic to it, but you would only find that out from trying it. Before you get carried away and rub it all over your body, patch test it on the back of your arm to see if you are allergic. You may notice some other problems: self-tanning creams can turn your skin a strange shade of orange, become patchy as the skin sheds, and build up unevenly on some areas of the body, such as knees, elbows, necks, and hands.

If you are willing to take your chances with a self-tanning cream, at least be sure to apply it evenly. Go slowly. Do not try to go from light to dark in a few days. Use very little of the product until you become adept at creating the look you want. If the cream begins turning your skin a strange shade of orange instead of golden brown, discontinue using it. The orange color isn't dangerous, only unattractive. Again, testing some of the cream on a small part of your body is a good way to find out if the tan color you get is the tan color you want. And what will inevitably happen to your semi-permanent tan when your skin sheds? Your skin will look extremely patchy and uneven because the self-tanning cream colors only the surface skin. Trying to put on more color may exaggerate the rough appearance. There is no easy answer, but if you are curious to see what happens to your skin, it may be worth a shot. For at least a week or two, it can look great.

All other fake tanning products now on the market, including those that are illegal, are potentially dangerous to use. Suntan pills are considered unsafe by the FDA and are being removed from the market. There are also repigmentation drugs available by prescription that contain an active ingredient called psoralen. This drug can be very effective for those people suffering from vitiligo, a skin disorder that leaves patches of skin void of color. But psoralen has serious side effects and it should never be used for the purpose of tanning.

What You Need to Know About All Moisturizers

Following is perhaps one of my most controversial opinions about skin care: if you don't have dry skin, you do not—I repeat, do not—need a moisturizer. If your skin is dry, you do need a moisturizer. All a moisturizer can do for you, to one extent or another, is retain moisture in the skin and smooth dry skin surfaces—no more and no less. If your oil glands are doing their job, you don't need a moisturizer. If your oil glands can't keep up with your dry skin, then you do need a moisturizer. Your skin will not wrinkle any faster if you don't use one. In fact, if you use a moisturizer when you don't really need one, you can end up with oily skin, clogged pores, whiteheads, blemishes, and a dull-looking skin surface. Overusing moisturizers can cause major skin problems. Your skin will actually fare much better if you don't load it up with unnecessary creams and lotions.

If you've made it this far, you now know that wrinkle creams are nothing more than moisturizers, and moisturizers are good for taking care of dry skin. All the other misleading and exaggerated claims about everything from firming or nourishing the skin to stimulating cellular regeneration can be ignored. Now we can focus on what moisturizers can do and which moisturizing ingredients to look for.

> If you use a moisturizer when you don't really need one, you can end up with oily skin, clogged pores, whiteheads, blemishes, and a dull-looking skin surface.

A good moisturizer can quite nicely take care of dry skin. The type of moisturizer you need depends on how dry your skin is. Almost every moisturizer on the market—yes, I said almost every moisturizer on the market—regardless of price, brand name, or fancy claims, can benefit the skin by counteracting the effects of dry skin. Are there differences among moisturizers? Yes. Are some better than others? Most definitely. But all moisturizers are capable of improving dry skin. How well a moisturizer can do that depends on what's in it and not the price or fancy claims. Which ingredients should you look for, not which moisturizer should you select, is the question that needs answering.

How Moisturizers Do What They Do

There are two major ways moisturizers work to soothe dry skin and prevent loss of water from the skin. One way is by stopping the air from absorbing the water from the skin into the atmosphere. The air can remove the water from the face the same way it absorbs water from the ground. The drier the climate, the harsher the weather, or the more dry heat you are exposed to, the drier your skin can be. Using a moisturizer that can keep the air off your face is very important. Using one that can hold water in the skin for longer periods of time is equally important. There are two groups of moisturizing ingredients that work toward accomplishing these two tasks for the skin, and you need to become familiar with them.

Good moisturizers contain oils (or ingredients that act like oils on the surface of the skin) that can keep the air off the face and ingredients that can hold or bind water to the skin for longer periods of time. For the most part, oils smooth over the top of the skin and form a barrier to prevent the air from drinking up the water in the skin cell. The oil in your moisturizer literally replaces the oil your oil glands are not providing for you. When you buy a moisturizer you want to be sure you are purchasing one that contains some type of oil. Water-binding ingredients come in a few different forms, but they all pretty much do the same thing; that is, they keep water in the skin.

Which oils and water-binding ingredients are the best? That is an excellent question. Basically there are four types of oils found in moisturizers: vegetable, mineral, animal (fats), and vitamin E oils. There are also a handful of ingredients that act like oil on the skin and bind water to the skin: collagen, proteins, amino acids, and mucopolysaccharides. This group does an excellent job of keeping the air off the face *and* holding water in the skin.

Vegetable oils. Dozens of vegetable oils are used in moisturizers, among them avocado, sweet almond, sunflower, jojoba, safflower, basil, corn, coconut, sandalwood, wheat germ, rice bran, olive, macadamia, palm, carrot, peach, grape seed, soybean, and castor oil. Is one better than the other? For the most part, all vegetable oils are pretty much created equal and function beautifully to help dry skin retain water. Any of these vegetable oils is a good ingredient to have in a moisturizer designed for dry skin. The benefit of a vegetable oil is that some of it can be absorbed into the lower layers of skin and protect the skin cells under the surface.

There is a problem with using vegetable oils in cosmetics because they turn rancid quite easily. The rancidity doesn't lessen the oil's effectiveness, but it does affect the way the cosmetic smells. There is no reliable way to prevent that from happening, so cosmetics that contain vegetable oils almost always contain fragrance to cover up the rancid smell. In spite of this problem with spoiling, vegetable oils are still desirable in creams and lotions designed for dry skin—that is, if you are not allergic to fragrance.

Mineral oils. There are two basic kinds of mineral oil—those derived from petrolatum (better known as Vaseline) and those derived from a group of ingredients called silicones such as dimethicone and cyclomethicone. (On a cosmetic ingredient label when mineral oil is listed it refers to the liquid version of petrolatum.) Mineral oil and petrolatum are very common moisturizing ingredients, and for two good reasons. First, they are very inexpensive, and second, they work. Petrolatum and mineral oil do not absorb into the skin because the molecules are too large to penetrate the skin. Therefore they stay on the surface of the skin and provide an occlusive barrier between the skin and the air. That is a good reason to look for mineral oil and petrolatum listed in a moisturizer. The same is true for the silicones, which also do an impressive job of keeping water in the skin by creating a strong barrier between the face and the air.

I should mention that some beauty experts feel that mineral oils are a skin care no-no and should be avoided at all costs. They feel they can cause blemishes and damage the surface of the skin. There are many moisturizing ingredients that can cause blemishes, so I'm not sure why these experts pick on mineral oil any more than, say, lanolin or vegetable oil, which are also known to clog pores and cause allergic reactions. I have not found enough supporting evidence to warrant avoiding any kind of mineral oil if you're not allergic to it. Besides, you are more likely to be allergic to a lot of other cosmetic ingredients than you are to mineral oil: lanolin, fragrance, perservatives, and alcohol, just to name a few. Although I recommend mineral oil, if you are concerned about it, there are plenty of substitute ingredients (listed in this section) that work very well.

Animal oils. Lanolin and fish oils are the typical animal fats you find in moisturizers. Research indicates that good old-fashioned lanolin is still the best ingredient for keeping water in the skin. The reason for this is that lanolin closely resembles the oil produced by human oil glands. For very dry skin, lanolin is an excellent moisturizing ingredient. The only negative is that lanolin can cause allergic reactions in some people. Unless your skin is sensitive to lanolin, there is no reason whatsoever to avoid it. Like vegetable oils, lanolin can penetrate the skin and protect the lower layers of skin cells.

There is another group of animal oils (fats) used in cosmetics found naturally in the skin. The most typical are cholesterol, glycolipids, and phospholipids. They are not exactly typical oils, but they work in a similar fashion to oils, keeping water in the skin and smoothing the outer and lower layers of skin cells. These lipids can be absorbed into the skin and work well as moisturizing ingredients.

Vitamin E. Vitamin E oil is a unique oil that is listed on cosmetic ingredients labels as tocopherol, its chemical name. (Cosmetic ingredients labels must list all vitamins by their chemical name so as not to mislead the consumer into thinking there is any nutrient value in the product.) Vitamin E has no miraculous properties, even though a lot of cosmetics companies would like you to believe it does. The latest claims about vitamin E stems from its supposed ability to keep free radicals off the face. There is no evidence that supports this claim, other than from cosmetics companies who want to sell you products that contain vitamin E. Nevertheless, vitamin E is still a good oil for the skin, much like all the other oils I've listed here. Vitamin E can cause allergic reactions for people with sensitive skin, but if you are not allergic to it, it is just fine. Vitamin E can be absorbed into the skin and protect the lower layers of skin cells.

Note: *These various types of oils are all beneficial for taking care of dry skin. Is one better than another? Not really. They all have their positives (keeping water in the skin) and negatives (possible allergic reactions). Cosmetics companies use various combinations of all these ingredients, particularly the more popular ones, to be sure the consumer won't be disappointed. Which combination of ingredients works best for your skin is best discovered by trying different products that include some of these oils or any of the ingredients I've listed in this section.*

Proteins. Collagen, other proteins, amino acids, hyaluronic acid, and mucopolysaccharides are all ingredients that form a film over the face and help prevent the skin from losing water. We all know by now that the collagen found in moisturizers cannot affect or change the collagen in our skin. It keeps moisture in the skin, but no better than any of the other ingredients listed in this section. Collagen is a worthwhile moisturizing ingredient because it doesn't absorb into the skin; it smoothes over the surface of the skin and keeps the air off the face. The same is true for other proteins, amino acids, hyaluronic acid, and mucopolysaccharides. These four types of ingredients are all related. Amino acids combine to make proteins; proteins combine to make mucopolysaccharides; and hyaluronic acid is a mucopolysaccharide. All of them have too large a molecular structure to be absorbed into the skin, so, much like mineral oils, they form a protective barrier over the face and help prevent dehydration. These water-binding ingredients are good to have in your moisturizer.

> You want to be sure the good ingredients are listed first.

Note: *Why not just use pure vegetable oil, mineral oil, lanolin, or vitamin E on your dry skin? There isn't actually anything wrong with doing that, and many women do. In fact, women who suffer from severely dry skin can benefit from using pure oils (even those right out of your kitchen cabinet) over the drier areas of the face. The problem with doing this is that using pure oil during the daytime will look fairly greasy and make makeup application almost impossible. At night pure oils are messy to sleep with and can smell bad.*

Summary:

The best moisturizers on the market contain at least one water-binding ingredient to keep water in the skin, a mineral oil to prevent air from drying up the water from the skin's surface, and one or more vegetable or animal oils to protect the lower layers of skin. What you will find is that many moisturizers (though definitely not all) meet these basic requirements.

The ingredients to avoid in moisturizers are fragrance, coloring agents, and preservatives, particularly when these ingredients are listed high up in the ingredients listing. Fragrance and coloring agents can cause allergic reactions in a lot of women. When preservatives are high up in the ingredients listing (instead of at the very end of the list) it indicates that a large amount of preservatives is being used, which can increase the chances of an allergic reaction. The other problem with preservatives, fragrance, and coloring agents being listed before the oils or other moisturizing ingredients listed above is that this order means that not much of the beneficial ingredients is present. You want to be sure the good ingredients are listed first.

Directions: *Apply the moisturizer over a clean face that is slightly damp. Do not rub the moisturizer into the face; that stretches and irritates the skin. Smooth the moisturizer evenly over the face and allow it to be absorbed into the skin. You do not need to use bottled or canned European water on your face. These pricey atomizers offer nothing special that cannot be simulated by wetting the fingers with tap water and dabbing the face or putting tap water into your own spray bottle and misting your face. Making this simple step more complicated and costly is one more way the cosmetics industry collects your money without providing a valuable product.*

What About Oil-Free Moisturizers?

Oil-free moisturizers are a curious assortment of products. They are almost always recommended to women who have oily skin or who tend to break out. You are supposed to believe that women with oily skin still need moisture in their skin, and therefore using a moisturizer is vital. None of that is true. If the skin is not dry, it does not require more moisture because it already has enough. Oil-free moisturizers are totally unnecessary if you don't have dry skin. If a woman who has oily skin is not doing anything to irritate or dry her face, it would be almost impossible for her to have dry skin. Unless you have dry skin, there is no need to bother with a moisturizer of any kind—never mind oil-free.

Oil-free is also a misleading term. Oil-free generally refers to a product that doesn't contain mineral oil, vegetable oil, or lanolin. There are many ingredients in moisturizers, particularly oil-free moisturizers, that don't have an "oily" sounding name but have the same effect as oil on the skin—which is precisely what oily skin does not need, more oil. The other problem is that many of these oil-free moisturizers are sold to women with mild acne under the pretense that they will not make them break out. There isn't a moisturizer invented that won't make most oily skins worse and encourage breakouts.

Can There Ever Be Enough Water?

Oils, proteins, and collagen work on the skin to prevent dehydration, and that is the only way they can keep water in the skin. If there isn't much water in the skin to start with, those ingredients just soothe the skin and do little else. The goal is to give the skin back some of the water it has lost and hold it in the skin for as long as possible. It would be nice if simply drinking more water could do that, but it can't. Drinking more water than the body needs simply would create more of a need to go to the bathroom.

One of the ways you can get extra water to your dry skin cells is to spray or dab the face with a light layer of water and then apply your moisturizer directly over the water. There is also some benefit to using a relatively new cosmetic ingredient called a liposome that is distinct from all the ingredients mentioned above. (Liposomes come in a wide variety of cosmetic names such as nanosomes, niosomes, and biosomes.)

Liposomes work on the skin much like timed-release vitamins or hayfever pills work in your body. Timed-release medications allow you to take one pill that lasts over a long period of time. Once swallowed, the chemicals are slowly released into the bloodstream. This way, the capsule's entire contents are not dumped into the body all at once, to be used up quickly, requiring you to take more in order to sustain the pill's benefits. Now imagine that timed-release effect waiting for you inside a moisturizer. Liposomes hold the oil and water from the moisturizer under the skin so they are not absorbed or wiped off. What that means is that you can't wash away the liposomes, or the water and oil attached to them, even after you wash your face. (The liposomes with their portion of water and oil are used up when the skin cell finally absorbs it.)

> The water that is absorbed into the skin cell will only stay there for as long as the oil stays around.

When you put on a moisturizer each of the ingredients has a particular destiny. Some of the mineral oil spreads over the surface of the skin and some of the vegetable or animal oils are absorbed into the skin. A very small amount of the water in the product spreads over the surface of the face and an even smaller portion of that is absorbed into the skin. (Most of the water in a moisturizer is never absorbed into the skin because it is absorbed by the air before it has a chance to go anywhere else.) The water that is absorbed into the skin cell will only stay there for as long as the oil stays around. As anyone with dry skin will attest, sometimes that isn't all that long. The mineral oil on the surface of the skin is easily wiped away during the day, and the vegetable or animal oils are eventually absorbed completely. The effects derived from wearing a moisturizer last only as long as the moisturizer is present. Liposomes can keep the moisturizer around for a longer period of time than is normal. How much longer is open to debate, but longer is considered a sure thing.

There are more and more products on the market that contain liposomes. L'Oréal, Lancôme, and Christian Dior all have several moisturizers that contain liposomes. Another, much more reasonably priced product, available at the drugstore, is called Candermyl. Candermyl is made by Alcon Laboratories in Fort Worth, Texas.

Special Waters

Many cosmetics companies tout their products as containing unique and amazing water such as *water dm*, sterilized water, ionized water, water from glaciers, or water from special mineral springs from some exotic locale. The claims are unsubstantiated by any independent, reliable sources. To put it simply, there is no difference between regular water and fancy water on the skin. Even if these claims were somewhat valid, all water used in cosmetics must be sterilized. Once water is purified at high temperatures and then added to a cosmetic filled with preservatives, whatever special properties the water was supposed to have had in the first place would all be boiled down to plain water. Even if the properties of the special water remained intact after the product was finally put together, the skin cell doesn't need and can't use "special" water.

Speaking of water, when you see aloe vera listed among the first ingredients in a cosmetic, realize that the aloe vera is nothing more than water. Aloe vera is only the juice from an aloe plant. The pure juice straight out of the plant might have some cooling benefit on the skin and marginal moisturizing ability, but from a chemical point of view it is 99.5 percent water and 0.5 percent protein. Whatever you want to believe about the 0.5 percent protein is up to you, but once the aloe vera is sterilized and placed in a cosmetic product, it is nothing more than water.

Ingredients in Moisturizers That Don't Work

I'm going to make this section short and sweet. There are many moisturizing ingredients that are worthwhile and extremely beneficial for the skin, and there are many ingredients that are useless and ineffective. In fact, many of the so-called miracle ingredients are not only ludicrous but downright laughable. My favorite example is a product by La Prairie called Essence of Skin Caviar that sells for $75 per half-ounce. What do you think could be in a product that retails for over $2,400 a pound? Except for placental protein, all the other ingredients are fairly standard moisturizing ingredients. The placental protein isn't even at the top of the ingredients list—it's at the bottom, which means it is the smallest-quantity ingredient in the jar.

What is placental protein? A piece of an animal's afterbirth. You are supposed to believe that a hunk of some animal's afterbirth mixed into your night cream is going to change your skin. Other companies claim that their products contain human placenta extract. The list goes on and on. "Spleen extract," from a dead cow's spleen, is supposed to smooth wrinkles, and "neural lipid extract," dead brain tissue, is supposed to be the key to flawless skin. The brain, spleen, and placenta extracts are only a representation of how absurd the cosmetics industry can get when trying to find ingredients that will turn you on. The other crazy ingredients that belong on this list are sea algae extract, amniotic fluid, animal thymus extract, animal tissue extract, epidermal lipid extract, serum albumin, serum protein, tissue matrix extract, cross-linked elastin, milk protein, royal bee jelly, vitamin A, retinyl palmitate, and retinol. (These last three ingredients are added to products so you believe you are getting something that will act like Retin-A on the skin. They won't.)

This list will keep on growing. As fast as one miracle shows up, another one from a different company can't be far behind. There are so many cosmetics miracles, it is amazing that any of us still has a wrinkle left— or a cent in our pockets.

Exotic Formulations?

Here's a good question. If all moisturizers are predominantly water, oil, and water-binding ingredients that act like oils, then why don't moisturizers look like a mixture of oil and water? Why do moisturizers, if they have so much in common, look and feel so different? The answer is because of the various forms of waxes that are used to give cosmetics their texture and appearance. This waxy group of ingredients comes in a multitude of forms that can be either *synthetic*, such as by-products from the manufacturing of alcohol or petroleum, or *natural*, as in waxes such as beeswax or ceresin. ades of waxes. Waxes thicken a moisturizer. They also help keep it stable and give the cream its texture and form. Different blends of waxes do not resemble each other. That is why even though the basic ingredients in moisturizers tend to be more or less the same, they do not always look the same or feel the same. But wax has no beneficial moisturizing effect.

The kind of texture you prefer in a moisturizer is a personal thing. What feels comfortable and soothing for your skin is what is best for you. There is nothing inherent in the texture of a moisturizer that makes it any better than any other at keeping water in the skin. The other ingredients—the oils and water-binding ingredients in combination—are the most important things to look for.

The Basic Skin Care Routine

Now that you have all the information about cleansers, scrub products, toners, facial masks, moisturizers, and wrinkle creams, the next step is to put the right combination together for each skin type. The basic skin care routine is as follows:

1 Twice a day, wash your face with a water-soluble cleanser, using tepid water. The cleanser I recommend is Cetaphil Lotion, which is available in most drugstores. Avoid bar soap and wipe-off makeup removers. The water-soluble cleanser will remove your eye makeup at the same time you wash your face. Tepid water is important because hot water burns and irritates the skin and cold water shocks and irritates it. Do not rub the skin dry with a towel; rather, gently blot it dry. Never pull at the skin. Any trace of eye makeup left behind can be removed with a cotton swab and the Cetaphil Lotion or your moisturizer. (Yes, your moisturizer can remove traces of leftover makeup.)

2 At night only, after the cleanser is rinsed off, while your face is still wet, massage your face with a blend of baking soda and water. If you have oily skin and breakouts you can use the baking soda mixed with water all over the face every night. If you have dry skin, mix the baking soda with Cetaphil Lotion or your water-soluble cleanser two to three times a week. Always massage gently and rinse very well. Do not overscrub. If you have extremely sensitive skin, massage the baking soda only over blemishes or areas where you break out. Remember to rinse well. Do not leave baking soda on the face. *Be careful*— you can overdo the baking soda.

3 If you have skin that has blemishes and/or blackheads, apply three percent hydrogen peroxide solution to those areas with a cotton ball twice a day. Let this dry. Avoid the hairline and the eyebrow area with the three percent hydrogen peroxide solution; the hair will lighten with repeated exposure. If you have sensitive skin, use a cotton swab to apply the three percent hydrogen peroxide solution only over specific blemishes, avoiding all other areas of the skin.

4 If you have dry or normal skin or do not have blemishes, you can use an irritant-free toner all over your face after the cleanser is rinsed.

5 For skin with blemishes or oily skin, use a facial mask of plain milk of magnesia two to three times a week depending on how oily the skin is. If you're not breaking out, then it is not necessary to use the milk of magnesia or the three percent hydrogen peroxide solution. If you have extremely sensitive skin and have breakouts, apply the milk of magnesia only over the blemishes and nowhere else. If your skin is normal, using the milk of magnesia is not necessary, but it won't hurt the skin if you enjoy applying a facial mask once in a while.

6 At night, if your skin is dry, moisturize your face by spraying it first with a light mist of water and then spreading your moisturizer over the water and letting it be absorbed into the skin. If you need to, you can dab off the excess. Do not rub or massage the moisturizer into your skin. The idea is to let it be absorbed. If your skin is not dry, you do not need a moisturizer.

7 During the day, for all skin types, use either a moisturizer or a foundation that contains a sunscreen of SPF 15 or greater. Many sunscreens contain the same ingredients as your favorite moisturizer, so you will not need both a sunscreen and a separate moisturizer during the day. If your face can't handle a sunscreen on a daily basis, do your best to avoid the sun as much as possible.

8 Regardless of the weather, use a sunscreen of SPF 15 or greater on all exposed parts of your body if you are planning to spend the day outside. When exercising or swimming, be sure to reapply your sunscreen every two to three hours, even if you are using a waterproof sunscreen.

9 If you have extremely dry skin, at night only, after you've applied your moisturizer, you can apply pure lanolin (you can buy this at the drugstore), pure vitamin E oil (you can find this at most health food stores), or any pure oil that you have in your kitchen over the parched areas of your face instead of expensive eye creams, which generally contain these same ingredients.

10 See your dermatologist if you're interested in trying Accutane for acne or Retin-A for acne and/or sun-damaged skin. There are no products on the market that can be substi-

tuted for these prescription drugs, regardless of the claims on the package.

ll Be sure to remove all your makeup every night and never sleep with your makeup on. Makeup left on overnight becomes an irritant on the face, prevents skin cells from shedding, and can clog pores. Swollen eyes, blackheads, dry patches, and rashlike blemishes can often be traced to leaving makeup on for longer than necessary. Give your face a rest and let your face breathe; your pores and skin will thank you.

The Best Skin Care Routine for Each Skin Type

Basic normal skin: Clean the face with a water-soluble cleanser twice a day. Use baking soda as a scrub mixed with your cleanser twice a week at night only. After you've cleansed your face both morning and night, use an irritant-free toner all over your face. During the day use a foundation or a light-feeling sunscreen with an SPF of 15 or greater. If your skin does not feel dry at night, you do not need to use a moisturizer.

Mature normal skin: Follow the same routine as for basic normal skin, except that if your skin is feeling drier at night than it has in the past, you will want to use a moisturizer. The moisturizer should not be greasy or rich. It is best to stay with a lightweight one and use that all over.

Basic oily skin: Clean your face twice a day with a water-soluble cleanser. If you feel your face needs more cleansing action to remove your makeup at night, wash it only with a water-soluble cleanser that has a slight amount of lather or with a gentle bar soap. In the morning wash your face with Cetaphil Lotion, which will leave the face feeling soft and not dry. At night, after the cleanser is rinsed off, use baking soda mixed with water directly on the face four to five times a week. Twice a day go over the areas of your face that tend to break out with three percent percent hydrogen peroxide solution (this is in place of a toner or an astringent). You can use a facial mask of milk of magnesia once a week. At night you do not need to use any moisturizers, including so-called oil-free moisturizers. During the day you should also avoid using all moisturizers. It is best for your skin type to use an oil-free foundation that contains a sunscreen of SPF 15 or greater.

Severely oily skin: Follow the same routine as for basic oily skin, except that you may want to try using the baking soda as a scrub morning and night. During the day, mix the baking soda with your water-soluble cleanser; at night you can still use it directly on the face. Use the milk of magnesia as a facial mask three to four times a week. At night never use a moisturizer of any kind unless you need one occasionally around the eye area, and then only use the tiniest amount. The same is true for daytime—do not use a moisturizer of any kind. It is best for your skin type to use an oil-free foundation that contains a strong sunscreen.

Mature oily skin: Depending on how oily your skin is, follow the guidelines for basic or severely oily skin. The only difference for your skin is that nowadays there may be dryness under the eye area. At night and before you put on your makeup, place a lightweight moisturizer under the eye area. If you have some dry skin, use your moisturizer over those areas only.

Acned oily skin: Follow the same guidelines as for basic oily skin. Be sure to go over the blemished areas an extra time with the three percent hydrogen peroxide solution. Place a small amount of the milk of magnesia over a blemish, let it dry, and then apply your foundation.

Acned dry skin: Wash your face twice a day with a water-soluble cleanser such as Cetaphil Lotion. At night massage only those areas that are breaking out with the baking soda mixed with your water-soluble cleanser, and rinse well. Twice a day use a cotton swab to soak only the blemishes with three percent hydrogen peroxide solution. You may follow this with an irritant-free toner over the entire face after the three percent hydrogen peroxide solution dries. If, after the irritant-free toner is applied, your face still feels dry, apply only a lightweight moisturizer that does *not* contain lanolin, isopropyl myristate, petrolatum, beeswax, cholesterol, or any other thick-feeling ingredients. During the day, after the irritant-free toner has dried, apply a lightweight foundation designed for normal to dry skin that contains a strong sunscreen. It is probably best to avoid a moisturizer during the day if your skin can handle it. Foundations designed for normal to dry skin may contain enough moisturizing ingredients to take care of your dry skin during the day.

Cystic acne: For this skin type it is best that you consult your dermatologist. Cosmetic skin care routines cannot really help.

Basic dry skin: Twice a day wash with Cetaphil Lotion or a similar water-soluble cleanser. Twice a week massage the skin with a mixture of baking soda and Cetaphil Lotion, and rinse well. Twice a day apply an irritant-free toner all over your face. During the day use a lightweight moisturizer with an SPF of 15 or greater over the face. At night, a richer creamlike moisturizer can be used all over the face.

Mature dry skin: Follow the recommendations for basic dry skin. There is essentially no difference between basic dry skin and mature dry skin except the texture, which has more impact on makeup application than it does on skin care.

Sensitive skin: Depending on what other skin type is present at the same time, you will want to be careful about how you use the baking soda and the three percent hydrogen peroxide solution. Other than that, Cetaphil Lotion, irritant-free toner, and lightweight or rich moisturizers should not cause you a problem unless you are allergic to the individual product you've chosen. Sensitive-skin types usually need to search more for products their skin can tolerate.

Combination skin: Avoid products that can aggravate the present skin types. For example, if you have oily skin that breaks out and dry skin, do not use the baking soda or the three percent hydrogen peroxide solution directly over the dry skin. Spot-using them where you have problems would be better. Also, avoid using your moisturizer over the areas where you have oily skin. If you have dry skin and oily skin in the same areas, then you are either using harsh products that I have not recommended or you are overdoing the baking soda and three percent hydrogen peroxide solution or milk of magnesia and need to cut back.

Note: *If you have a problem with eczema-like patches of dry skin or irritation on your face that persist regardless of how much moisturizer you use, especially if you've been using the water-soluble cleanser and irritant-free toner, you can purchase one of the over-the-counter hydrocortisone creams and see how that works for you. Apply the cream after you use your moisturizer and only over the irritated areas. If this doesn't help, you may want to consult a dermatologist who could prescribe a more potent cortisone cream for those problem areas.*

The Best Skin Care Products

This section briefly summarizes the information I wrote about extensively in my book *Don't Go to the Cosmetics Counter Without Me*. For the sake of review I will include the basic list here.

Water-soluble cleansers: Cetaphil Lotion is my favorite, but there is also Clean & Clear for Sensitive Skin by Revlon and Neutrogena's Facial Cleansing Formula. Eucerin Foaming Face Wash lathers more, but it can leave some skin types feeling a bit dry.

Bar soaps: Aveeno dry skin formula, Pears Soap, Dove and Neutrogena soap for dry skin only.

Scrubs: Baking soda is by far the best.

Toners: My favorite irritant-free toners are The Body Shop's Orange Flower Water and Honey Water, Borghese's Tonico Minerale, Chanel's Lotion Douce, Christian Dior's Skin Freshener, Clinique's Alcohol-free Clarifying Lotion, Estée Lauder's Gentle Protection Tonic, L'Oréal's Floral

Tonic, Physician's Formula Gentle Refreshing Toner, and Ultima II's CHR Extraordinary Gentle Clarifier.

Moisturizers: There are literally thousands of moisturizers on the market in all price ranges. Although it may sound a bit surprising, I really don't have a favorite. I encourage you to look first for ingredients and then texture, which can only be judged by testing it for yourself. To get you started, this is a list of my favorites that are also reasonably priced: Candermyl (for liposomes), Lubriderm, Nutraderm, Nivea Visage, L'Oréal's Plenitude line, and Revlon's European line.

Sunscreens: There are so many good ones out there that it is important only that you find one that feels good, and you won't know that until you try it. You may want to try the sunscreens sold by Nivea, Johnson & Johnson, Mary Kay, Clinique, or any other as long as they have an SPF of 15 or greater.

Reading the Ingredients Label with Confidence

The entire subject of cosmetics ingredients is a book all by itself and one that, although interesting, will possibly either bore you or totally confuse you. Cosmetic chemistry is a complicated, highly technical field of study. To impart some of that knowledge is not an easy task, especially if I want you to stay awake for the rest of the book. What may be helpful to you is listing a few rules and suggestions about how to understand the only part of cosmetics packaging that has any real meaning at all. As you get more familiar with the ingredients I've mentioned in the skin care section, you'll find that the following guidelines will help you even further.

1 Ingredients listings are legally controlled by the Food and Drug Administration.

2 Every cosmetic and pharmaceutical product—every one— must have a complete ingredients list that includes every chemical (natural or synthetic) that is used in the product. If the ingredients listing is not on the container itself, it will be on its package. At most cosmetics counters you have to ask for the packaging that has the label attached to it. Do not ever examine or choose to purchase a cosmetic again before you have read the ingredients list. Even if you do not understand the more technical-sounding names of the ingredients (and who does besides chemists anyway?), you can still become familiar with some of the basics that are in practically every product. There are many cosmetics ingredients that are easily decipherable

such as water, mineral oil, petrolatum, beeswax, vegetable oil, lanolin, glycerin, collagen, plant and food derivatives, talc, fragrance, and coloring agents. The more you can read an ingredients list, the less mysterious cosmetics will be to you.

3 The most important thing to remember is that all cosmetics ingredients are listed in descending order. The first ingredient is the most abundant (probably more than 70 percent of the product's content) and the last ingredient is the least present (probably less that 0.5 percent of the product's content). When you are trying to find good moisturizing ingredients you want them to be among the first in the list, not the last. If it's a good product, the special ingredients will be up front.

4 Long ingredients listings do not necessarily mean the product has a more exotic formulation. I have heard from more than one dermatologist that a long cosmetics ingredients list should be treated with concern. One reason for this is that the more complicated the listing, the more likely you are to find something in there that you're allergic to. Simple listings of good ingredients are more impressive to me than long ones.

5 The part of the label you can ignore with confidence is the description of what the product can do. Almost without exception this is not going to help you make an informed decision. This is what the cosmetics company *wants* you to believe. That a product *nourishes the skin, plumps the skin, smooths cellulite, produces flawless skin,* or *stops oil production* are not claims you need to give credence to any longer. Also, many labels that say the product is noncomedogenic falsely imply that the product does not contain ingredients that can make the skin break out.

6 Do not be confused or misled by exotic-sounding ingredients —the way something sounds is not necessarily the way it is.

7 When it comes to skin care products, consider looking only for products that do not contain fragrance or coloring agents. It is also a good idea to buy cosmetics that list the preservatives last. The names of the most widely used preservatives are methylparaben, propylparaben, butylparaben, ethylparaben, methylisothiazolinone, imidazolidinyl urea, diazolidinyl urea, dehydroacetic acid (DHA), BHT, BHA, quaternarium-1 through -7, quaternarium-8 through -15, quaternary ammonium compounds, trisodium EDTA, and disodium EDTA. The fewer of these in your cosmetic, the less likely it is that you will have an allergic reaction to it.

8 There is an excellent book on the market that deals exclusively with the subject of cosmetics ingredients—called *A Consumer's Dictionary of Cosmetic Ingredients* by Ruth Winter, published by Crown Publishers, Inc. I recommend this book wholeheartedly if you really want to understand what almost every ingredient in your cosmetics is for. This book isn't for everyone—it isn't what I would call engaging reading—but it is a must for the truly shrewd, patient cosmetics shopper.

Comparison Shopping for Skin Care Products

When you do go shopping for skin care products, here are a few tips to keep in mind. Be aware that companies claim differences between products that often don't exist. On the surface they may indeed look different, but inside they can be quite similar. Comparing labels will help you find out if that's the case. For example, when comparing water-soluble cleansers, if oil is listed in the first five to seven ingredients you can be sure it will be tricky to rinse off without the aid of a washcloth.

Natural ingredients, or *medically tested or scientifically formulated cleansers,* as I explained earlier, sound like they're good for the skin, but those terms are all essentially meaningless. None of those things on the label reflects results, which brings me to the most important advice I can render: the bottom line when it comes to most skin care products—particularly moisturizers and cleansers—is that you need to try the product before you buy it. You can usually convince cosmetics salespeople to give you a small sample if you supply the container. A container can be anything from a piece of tinfoil to a plastic bag. Then at your leisure you can take it home and see if it works for you. You would be surprised at the number of samples most cosmetics salespeople have at their disposal for free giveaways. Do not hesitate to ask.

Allergic Reactions

Hypoallergenic is a scientific-sounding word with no legal basis. The same is true for *allergy-tested products.* Although the products may indeed have been allergy-tested, you have no way of knowing which allergies were tested or on whom these tests were performed. Dealing with individual allergic reactions to cosmetics takes more information than those useless phrases and terms could ever provide. Many allergic reactions are caused from a combination of products—your foundation mixed with an eyeshadow or your moisturizer worn under a new blush. It isn't always one particular item that could be causing you problems, and to make matters more complicated, emotions can play a major part in making your skin react. Your moisturizer and the fight you had with your husband could trigger a skin reaction. The next week, the same moisturizer minus the argument may produce no reaction. There is also an additional stumbling block that makes allergies a very frustrating experience. What you are not allergic to today, you may become allergic to tomorrow and vice versa.

Two of the most common irritants in any cosmetic are the fragrance and the preservative. Use fragrance-free moisturizers to avoid these problems. It is a bit trickier, if not impossible, to find products that are preservative free. You will want to be sure the preservatives are the last ingredients listed on the label. Other potential allergens are the irritants I've been referring to all along: alcohol, scrubs, strong detergents, menthol, and some natural ingredients like vitamins and oils such as vitamin E and peppermint. And remember, don't go to bed with makeup on.

If you are convinced that you had an allergic reaction to a particular product or even a group of products, return them. Most companies will refund your money. It is in your best interest, as well as the interest of the cosmetics companies, to know which of their products may be causing problems for the population as a whole. If you don't inform them, they won't know. When you bring the product in for a refund, if the salesperson tells you this has never happened before, either ask to speak to the manager or ask for the direct number to the company. You will not get stuck with a product that has caused you problems if you are insistent, direct, and honest.

Allergic reactions are not alway minor. If you have a severe reaction do not hesitate to consult your physician or go to a hospital emergency room. Your skin's health is very important.

Chapter Three
Retin-A from a New Perspective

Separating the Publicity from the Reality

There is no ingredient in all of cosmetics history that has elicited the fame and notoriety that retinoic acid (Retin-A) has. Several years have gone by since the publicity-crazed days when the first stories about Retin-A hit the airwaves. Every conceivable news medium in the United States, Canada, Australia, New Zealand, South Africa, England, Japan, and Europe ran articles, interviews, reviews, critiques, warnings, and praises about the prescription-only wrinkle cream known as Retin-A. That was more than four years ago. Now that the hoopla about Retin-A has calmed down a bit and the media has left Retin-A in the dust, we can perhaps talk about the subject a little more clearly than we could before.

The one thing about Retin-A that hasn't changed in the past four years is what it is. Retin-A is an acid that is created when vitamin A is broken down into smaller chemical groupings. Retin-A is an active ingredient and has some very potent effects on the skin. In the United States it is only available by prescription. The Food and Drug Administration has been considering approving Retin-A for over-the-counter use, but at this writing nothing has changed. Retin-A is still a drug, and many dermatologists think it should stay that way.

The research study supposedly demonstrating Retin-A's ability to erase wrinkles that was released to the media back in the winter of 1988 was paid for by—guess who—Johnson & Johnson, the pharmaceutical company that distributes Retin-A. Not what you would call an objective study. Also, this so-called landmark study tested Retin-A on only thirty subjects. It was not what you would call a far-reaching study. There were other problems with the study that left gaping holes in its reliability. There was no control group established against which to compare the results.

Of particular ridicule were the before-and-after pictures, which were blatantly misleading as a result of poor lighting and apparent cosmetic application used to demonstrate the test results. Regardless of all this questionable data, the news headlines continued for months and the sales of Retin-A doubled. It didn't seem to matter whether the data were weak or inconclusive or that there were no independent studies available to corroborate the original research. The publicity release sounded legitimate enough, and besides, who wants to look a gift horse in the mouth? If a dermatologist says he's found a wrinkle cream, who cares if he was paid by the company that makes the cream to say so? Although not legitimate by most research standards, the bottom line is that Retin-A sells. The question that still remains is, does Retin-A work? That is an excellent question.

After talking to hundreds of women and dermatologists, the overwhelming answer to the question about whether or not Retin-A works or doesn't work is yes, no, and maybe. Yes, it does seem to prevent some forms of skin cancer and it does seem to smooth and heal the outer layer of sun-damaged skin. No, it does not get rid of or reduce deep, embedded wrinkles. And it is not yet proven whether or not Retin-A can stimulate the growth of collagen and elastin in the dermis. The next question is, is Retin-A worth using? The answer is a resounding yes, no, and maybe.

Many dermatologists are skeptical about whether Retin-A can live up to even half of its claims. I am concerned that women might be expecting too much from any so-called wrinkle cream, whether it be Retin-A or a cosmetic cream. What is known for certain is that Retin-A is not the fountain of youth or even a close approximation. It has some wonderful properties and benefits, but it is not the wrinkle cream Johnson & Johnson would lead us to believe. In the long run, I do believe there are positives to be found in using Retin-A, but the expectations about and the realities of this drug need to come closer together. The next question is, who then should consider using Retin-A?

Who Should Use Retin-A?

Anyone with some amount of sun-damaged skin. How do you get sun-damaged skin? By spending many unprotected hours in the sun. What happens to your skin? The outer layer thickens; the lower layers thin; the skin can develop brown or ashen discolorations; facial blood vessels are damaged and blocked; collagen and elastin fibers are destroyed; the skin can grow small, thickened patches of raised skin; and the chances of getting skin cancer are increased drastically. The reason for using Retin-A is that a large percentage of women with some amount of sun-damaged skin, who can successfully use it, will probably experience some change in their sun-damaged skin (although relief from deep wrinkles is not one of the benefits), and they may protect themselves from developing some forms of skin cancer. That's not bad for one little tube of cream that sells for less then most fancy wrinkle creams at the cosmetics counters.

Having said all that, there is also a percentage of women who should not bother to use Retin-A in spite of the potentially positive results. Women with ultra-sensitive skin may find it impossible to use Retin-A on a regular basis, and using it regularly is the key to sucess. Part of the game plan when using Retin-A is making a commitment to it. Retin-A must be used on a routine basis in order for it to work. If you aren't sure you can follow through with the routine, getting a prescription for Retin-A will be a waste of time. Also, Retin-A is *not* for people who don't have sun-damaged skin, and it is definitely *not* for people who are unwilling to give up getting a tan. Besides the fact that continued tanning while using Retin-A negates its effect, one of the more negative aspects of using Retin-A is that the skin can become ultrasensitive to the sun. The likelihood of getting a sunburn increases manyfold.

The other thing to keep in mind about Retin-A is that it is a drug and not a cosmetic. You can't just rub Retin-A into the skin and forget about it; it isn't necessarily that easy. There are potentially negative side effects to this drug and warnings go along with using it. Knowing what the risks are will make your decision about using Retin-A an appropriate one. Plus, all this information can help you use Retin-A more successfully right from the very start.

Summary:

Retin-A can be a good alternative for those women who want to see a texture difference in their sun-damaged skin, but it won't eliminate wrinkles, and it does have some potentially negative side effects.

Retin-A Impostors

After the media onslaught about Retin-A, most cosmetics companies scrambled to jump on the bandwagon. No self-respecting cosmetics executive could let this kind of free publicity fall through the cracks. Everyone had to have Retin-A in their skin care formulas or they were destined to become dinosaurs. But cosmetics companies could not use Retin-A in their products. Retin-A is sold only by prescription in most countries, including the United States, Canada, Australia, and England. What could a cosmetics executive do? Of course! Use ingredients that sound like Retin-A and claim that they can do practically the same thing as Retin-A without any of the negative side effects. It doesn't matter if the medical community tells women that only Retin-A can work like Retin-A, because there will be plenty of women who won't believe them. The medical community has been telling women for years that wrinkle creams don't work, and millions of women still buy wrinkle creams.

Knowing that women would be swayed by the association of ingredients that sounded similar to Retin-A, cosmetics companies created a whole new generation of cosmetics gimmicks. The result is that cosmetics line after cosmetics line included one or more of the following ingredients in their moisturizers and wrinkle creams: retinyl palmitate, vitamin A, retinol, and palmitic acid. None of these ingredients can behave in any way, shape, or form like Retin-A, but that doesn't stop the claims one little bit. The salespeople for these Retin-A look-alikes will try to tell you otherwise. They will insist that some other less irritating, nonprescription form of Retin-A is hiding out in a particular product. They will point to the ingredients and tell you that the Retin-A impostors are almost exactly like the real thing. They are nothing like Retin-A, and for now there isn't anything else around anywhere that can substitute. Retin-A, by prescription only, is the Retin-A we are discussing.

Some people think that taking vitamin A in increased doses is an "oral" approach to reducing wrinkles. It does sound logical. Retin-A is a derivative of vitamin A: it seems logical to assume that taking vitamin A orally should do similar things to the skin as applying Retin-A topically. To some extent vitamin A can work on the skin from the inside out, but the negative side effects of large doses are dangerous. The maximum daily requirement for vitamin A is only 4,000 to 5,000 units. What happens when you take too much vitamin A is that it can build up in the liver and cause serious side effects, it can cause arthritic-type pain in the bones and joints, and it can cause fetal deformities. Retin-A, on the other hand, has no such negative side effects associated with it. Vitamin A and Retin-A are related, but only in name, not in effect.

Can Retin-A cause damage internally when applied to the surface of the skin? While millions of women of all ages have used Retin-A for over thirty years, there have been no documented side effects other than irritation. Is the irritation dangerous? No, just irritating, and it stops when you discontinue using the Retin-A or when your skin adjusts to it.

What about applying plain vitamin A to the surface of the skin? If vitamin A can be so potent orally, it should be able to do something to the surface of the skin, right? No. This was tried experimentally years ago and found to be completely useless. Again, it may sound logical, but in practice it was a waste of time and effort.

Retin-A—The Story

The story of Retin-A is less dramatic than one might expect from a cream that researchers say may possess the ability to alter the appearance of wrinkles and sun-damaged skin. You might have thought that Retin-A was some ingenious, mysterious compound developed in some secret lab in the Alps or Himalayas with an exotic, rare tropical root as its active ingredient, which would be wonderfully romantic and make great copy but would also be totally untrue. It all started more than twenty-five years ago in Philadelphia (a very exotic location) at the University of Pennsylvania with the guru of skin care himself, Dr. Albert M. Kligman.

Known for his bold, outspoken, and authoritative dermatologic research on acne and aging, Dr. Kligman had been successfully using a derivative of vitamin A, known as tretinoin or retinoic acid (Retin-A), for his patients with acne. After a period of time his older patients began noticing a startling improvement in the appearance of their skin. The texture of their skin seemed to have improved.

Dr. Kligman states that even he was skeptical at first. He assumed his patients were under some type of psychological illusion. Perhaps they were so happy and relieved when their skin cleared up that they simply perceived themselves as looking better and younger. That would hardly be a surprising emotional side effect. But that was not the case. Ten years later the comments from Dr. Kligman's patients about experiencing smoother skin persisted. This time Dr. Kligman started noticing the differences, too. As Dr. Kligman himself says, "I wish I could say it was creative genius, but it was just an accident."

Accident or not, a study was commissioned by Johnson & Johnson, the company that purchased from Dr. Kligman the rights to manufacture Retin-A, to prove its effect on sun-damaged skin. The research took place over a sixteen-week period with thirty participants. At the end of the research, twenty-six of the thirty participants who completed the study were said to have manifested a significant improvement on the areas of skin that were treated with Retin-A. The adverse reactions cited in this experiment were that 92 percent of the patients developed some degree of mild to severe dermatitis and a few had to drop out of the study due to serious skin irritation. The conclusions of this research were published in the *Journal of the American Medical Association*, which made it all sound very official and acceptable. As you already know, it was then enthusiastically reported all over the world. To say the least, Johnson & Johnson is one happy company, and so are its stockholders.

The part of this historical essay that is important to focus on is that Retin-A has been around a long time and the effects on the skin are intriguing and can be beneficial. I am, however, concerned and disturbed about how a minor scientific study got so blown out of proportion. I am also dismayed at the overstatements that have become attached to Retin-A. Hopefully, after reading all this, you will view the information from a less muddled, hyperbolic outlook.

Why is Retin-A Available by Prescription Only?

The first year or two that all this hullabaloo about using Retin-A as a wrinkle cream was going on, there was much talk about the Food and Drug Administration approving Retin-A as an over-the-counter pharmaceutical. There are many drug-type products available that do not require a prescription. Sunscreens with an SPF rating, some topical cortisone creams, aspirin, ibuprofen, acetaminophen, benzyl peroxide, and most cold medications are all drugs that are approved for sale without prescription. So why not Retin-A, too? There are a lot of politics that go into establishing how a drug becomes categorized as prescription only versus over-the-counter, but the major considerations of the FDA are the potential side effects of the drug, the need for monitoring those effects by a physician, and the number of tests needed to prove its safety and effectiveness.

The reason it is highly unlikely that Retin-A will have its status changed from prescription only to over-the-counter has to do with a potential side effect that is considered possible although highly unlikely. Retin-A is a tretinoid, which is the oral drug classification of all derivatives of vitamin A. When tretinoids are taken internally, they can cause fetal abnormalities. Although there have been no documented cases of fetal abnormalities from using topical Retin-A, the remote possibility does exist and should not be ignored. If you are pregnant, the decision to use Retin-A needs to be made with your physician and not on your own.

The entire question about what is a drug versus what is a cosmetic is actually quite controversial, at least from the perspective of the cosmetics industry. Federal legislation defines a drug as "an article for use in the diagnosis, cure, mitigation, treatment, or province of disease or intended to affect or change a structure of the body." Cosmetics are described as "articles for use intended to be applied to the body for cleaning, beautifying, promoting attractiveness, or improving the appearance." In this country, drugs are strictly controlled; cosmetics by comparison have little to no controls at all.

There is a big difference as to how much research a cosmetic has to go through before it comes to market and how much research a drug needs before it can be sold to the public. Cosmetics require *no* proof of any kind that they can do what they claim they do. A drug, however, requires years of expensive, substantiated research before it can be released mass market. Cosmetics claims often sound like the claims of a drug, but as long as the product is a cosmetic, there is no research needed to back up any of the things the label declares. That is no small detail. The fact that cosmetics do not have to verify their claims gives the cosmetics companies a wide berth. All the statements in those pretty brochures they give away at the cosmetics counters or on their packages do not have to be substantiated. The research does not have to be confirmed by anyone.

Cosmetics companies complain that it would cost them too much money to do the research necessary to have their wrinkle creams or moisturizers approved by the FDA. That is a great ruse. If their products really could do what they claim, then approval by the FDA would stimulate sales in much the same way it did for Retin-A (sales were doubled in the first three months after the research was published). Not much of a cost when you consider the promise of sales. But the cosmetics companies know their wrinkle creams can't pass muster, so why bother, especially when they don't have to. The lack of documentation hardly affects the consumer's desire for expensive, though useless, wrinkle creams. For the most part, the cosmetics companies take advantage of the lack of regulations required by the FDA for cosmetics.

Should You Use Retin-A?

After the news broke about Retin-A and its potentially dramatic effect on wrinkles caused by sun damage, many dermatologists who normally had been writing twenty prescriptions a month for Retin-A were writing about 200. Pharmacists all over the country could not keep Retin-A in stock. Thousands of women impulsively jumped on the Retin-A band-wagon and began requesting prescriptions from any doctor they could find who would write one up for them. Everyone from gynecologists to pediatricians and dentists were writing prescriptions for Retin-A. And why not? As far as most doctors were concerned, there were absolutely no serious side effects associated with Retin-A. The drug had been around for more than thirty years without any serious problems. The worst that could happen was that a woman would experience a little irritation, which would go away immediately once use was stopped. If a woman wanted to see if Retin-A could change her wrinkles, what could it hurt?

With prescription in hand, a quick stop at a pharmacy would get you at least a three-month supply of Retin-A for under $30. Then with tube in hand you could head home and commence applying the stuff all over your face. Now all you needed to do was remember to use it nightly and then wait patiently (or impatiently, depending on your expectations) to see the ravages of time's fury erased forever from your face. In about a week or two, while you were waiting, you would probably start experiencing inflamed, red, and dried-out skin. So much for expectations! (Nowadays most dermatologists know to start their patients with sun-damaged skin on a lesser strength of Retin-A, but that doesn't mean you still won't experience some potent skin problems before you see results.)

The major point to be made here is that before you do anything you will want to reevaluate all the information about Retin-A so you can make an informed decision about whether or not this treatment, with all its positives and negatives, is something you want. Once that has been done, you may then decide to give Retin-A a try—and you'll be prepared for the possible side effects. Although I understand the urgency of your wanting to get some of this stuff home as soon as possible, I also know what can happen when things like this are done haphazardly. Remember, an ounce of prevention can be worth a pound of smooth skin.

What Retin-A Really Does

Explaining what Retin-A really does is no easy task because there is so much disagreement about how it affects the skin—and not just a little disagreement, but radical differences of opinion. There are those dermatologists who will tell you that Retin-A can do just about everything short of a face-lift. They assert that Retin-A can: transform abnormal, sun-damaged skin cells back to normal ones; rebuild the collagen and elastin fibers of the skin; increase the cell turnover rate of the epidermis; eliminate a proportionate amount of sun-damaged skin's leathery texture; reduce fine lines and some deeper sun-induced lines; influence the production of blood vessels; change the yellow or ashy color of sun-damaged skin back to a brighter pigment; remove brown sun spots; and cure some forms of skin cancer. After hearing all this you would wonder why everyone isn't using Retin-A. The reason everyone is *not* using Retin-A is that not all of those claims are substantiated, and many (if not most) women who use Retin-A have not experienced all, or even some, of these claims.

On the other side of the Retin-A spectrum, a large number of dermatologists would disagree with the assessment of those claims and would suggest that only two, or possibly three, of them are valid. Aside from these differences, which I will explain in a moment, there is a consensus among experts. What all dermatologists agree on is that Retin-A can increase skin cell turnover and skin cell shedding; it can also repair sun-damaged skin cells and make the skin's surface look smoother. Almost all of the dermatologists I've interviewed felt there is some (or even a lot of) benefit to be derived from using Retin-A.

Retin-A can change abnormal skin cells back to normal. This includes sun-damaged skin cells as well as chronically dry skin cells, which also look misshapen under the microscope. But remember, abnormal skin cells, whether they are caused by the sun or by dry skin, have nothing to do with wrinkling. Wrinkling begins with the breakdown of collagen and elastin fibers in the lower layers of skin. That destruction is a separate process from the formation of healthy epidermal skin cells. However, when you have healthy, plump, evenly shaped skin cells, your skin's surface will have a smoother feel and appearance. Most women I interviewed felt that Retin-A did not change their wrinkles, but they almost all said their skin looked and felt somewhat smoother.

Can Retin-A rebuild or stimulate the production of collagen and elastin fibers of the skin? This point is much more controversial than any of the other questions concerning Retin-A. Most of the dermatologists I interviewed said they thought the answer was *probably not*. However, according to Dr. Kligman's research, Retin-A can help repair the collagen and elastin fibers in the skin. But the word *help* is an imprecise word, and this research finding can be exaggerated. It seems that collagen and elastin have the ability to repair themselves. It seems Retin-A may help speed up the repair process. What is considered highly *unlikely* is that Retin-A can generate the production of new collagen and elastin fibers. A good analogy for this is to a flat tire. A tire with a hole the size of your foot cannot be repaired, but a tire with a small hole the size of the tip of your finger can be repaired. If the collagen and elastin in your skin can be repaired, it is thought that Retin-A can help, but if the collagen and elastin are completely destroyed, there is little to no chance of generating brand-new fibers with the use of Retin-A. It is universally believed that once the collagen and elastin fibers are destroyed and a wrinkle has set in, Retin-A won't change it.

Can Retin-A increase the cell turnover rate of the epidermis? Without question, Retin-A can—and quite well, for that matter. But just how increased cell turnover is generated is not something with which everyone agrees. Retin-A irritates the skin, and this irritation, like all skin irritation, can stimulate cell growth. Moreover, Retin-A may also directly stimulate the production of new skin cells, but this is debatable. Nevertheless, it is agreed that Retin-A does help skin cell turnover and as a result can thicken the surface layers of skin with healthy skin cells. To what degree is also debatable.

Can Retin-A reduce the fine lines and some of the deeper sun-induced lines? Because Retin-A can increase skin cell turnover it can make some superficial wrinkles look diminished. Retin-A does not eliminate or reduce deep, sun-induced wrinkles, expression wrinkles, or sagging.

Can Retin-A influence the production of blood vessels? This is another controversial point. Many people experience a brighter glow to their face while using Retin-A. The assumption is that this has something to do with the creation of new capillaries in the dermis. There are no studies that substantiate this claim. The brighter glow to the face comes mostly from the irritation the Retin-A causes the skin.

Can Retin-A change the yellow or ashy color of sun-damaged skin to a brighter, more even pigment? Yes, to some extent it can. One of the things that causes sun-damaged skin to look ashy or yellow is the buildup of thicker skin. The thickness of the skin prevents the blood from circulating nearer the surface, reducing the color the blood flow brings to the face. Because Retin-A thins the surface layers of skin, the circulation is more apparent on the surface. Also, because the outer layer of skin has been thinned, less melanin will build up at the surface. This reduction in melanin helps the skin to regain some of its original color tone. How much of a change you can expect to see differs widely depending who you talk to. But there is a consensus that Retin-A can improve the color of the face.

Can Retin-A cure or prevent skin cancer? Because Retin-A can generate or stimulate the production of new, healthy, and normal skin cells and eliminate the thickened, misshapen, abnormal skin cells at the surface, it is believed that Retin-A can indeed prevent some forms of basal cell skin cancer. To what degree and how reliably it can do this is not agreed upon. This is one question about Retin-A that you would need to ask your doctor. Anything on your face or body that you think might be related to skin cancer must be immediately checked out by your doctor. Never use Retin-A for skin cancer prevention or treatment on your own.

Can Retin-A eliminate the presence of brown sun spots from the skin? There are many doctors who prescribe Retin-A for just this effect. It seems that much the same way Retin-A can smooth thickened patches of sun-damaged skin, it can also fade the melanin buildup of sun spots. Some people have claimed total elimination of this problem. How well it can work for you is unknown, but the potential seems encouraging.

Summary:

So what can Retin-A do? If your skin is sun-damaged, Retin-A can improve the texture of the skin's surface; increase cell production; reduce the appearance of fine, superficial, sun-damaged lines; improve color tone; diminish the appearance of pigmentation spots caused by sun damage; and reduce the presence of dry skin that is caused by repeated sun exposure. What can't Retin-A do? Retin-A cannot change or eliminate deep sun-damaged wrinkles, it cannot produce more blood vessels, and it cannot produce new collagen or elastin. What are some of the more questionable results to be obtained from using Retin-A? There are those who assert that Retin-A can rebuild the skin's structure back to a totally normal, non-sun-damaged state, that it can cure and prevent some forms of skin cancer, and that it can make the skin stronger and more resistant to bacteria and the elements.

Despite all the confusion and concerns revolving around Retin-A, it would be hard for anyone to ignore the advantages of using it. That doesn't mean we should all immediately make an appointment with a dermatologist; there are still a few more points to consider before you get involved with Retin-A.

What is the Irritation All About?

One of the properties of Retin-A is that it is an acid: retinoic acid to be specific, a derivative of vitamin A. The fact that Retin-A is an acid should be taken quite seriously. Acids—even mild ones—can burn the skin, and that is one of the things that happen when you begin to use Retin-A. The burning takes place both on the surface of the skin and underneath. The initial irritation created by the Retin-A is necessary for it to work and to create the beneficial changes. How much irritation should you expect? That depends on your skin's sensitivities, whether or not you keep other irritants off your skin, and what strength of Retin-A you start out using.

If all this talk about irritation seems like too much to put up with, I understand completely. It isn't the most fun I can think of. Makeup application can be difficult, and your skin can look rather flaky and dehydrated until it adjusts to the Retin-A. There is also the burning, tingling sensation on the skin that you must put up with, which is definitely bothersome. All of these things can be part of the bargain of using Retin-A. Before you decide to chuck this entire section on Retin-A, consider the notion that it is the only "wrinkle cream" on the market that makes a long-term difference to the skin.

Retin-A is not a fluffy cosmetic cream that makes vague promises and delivers nothing but temporary relief from dry skin. Retin-A changes the skin and can improve the status of sun-damaged skin. To what extent the skin changes is up for argument, but change it does, and that change is for the better. The irritation is not great, but the irritation does go away, and what you will be left with is smoother skin.

I've mentioned a few times now that the irritation and dryness that are caused by using Retin-A will go away after the skin adjusts to it. How soon can you expect the irritation and dryness to go away? There is no set answer for this one. Some people experience no irritation, while others experience extreme reactions. Judging from the experiences of the dermatologists I've interviewed and my own, the average length of time for the irritation and dryness to persist is about two to four months, and then, it seems, the skin problems disappear.

There are ways to combat the dryness and irritation associated with Retin-A, but I'll talk about that more in the next few sections.

Does Retin-A Work for Everyone?

Retin-A is not for everyone, nor does it work the same way on all skin types. Initial studies indicate that the more advanced the sun damage, the less effect Retin-A will have. This is a drug that is better thought of as being preventive as opposed to curative or corrective. If you've been sunning your skin for decades, and sometime around the age of fifty or sixty you decide to start using Retin-A, the likelihood is that you will not see much of a change in your skin. Damage that advanced would take years or decades of using Retin-A to repair.

The most beneficial age to start seems to be in the late twenties to early thirties. If the skin is only somewhat sun-damaged by then, it is easier to restore. It seems Retin-A works slowly over time, and if the damage is too far gone, Retin-A can't do that much. This doesn't mean there is no benefit to be had if you start later in life, but the best age, according to Dr. Kligman, is younger as opposed to older.

I should mention that there is some controversy regarding this notion of when to start Retin-A. The question is, does the benefit from using Retin-A when you are younger come from using the Retin-A or from having skin that's been less exposed to the sun? If you do not build up years of damage on the skin, then it isn't the Retin-A that worked, but being exposed less to the sun. There is no absolute answer to this one yet, but for those dermatologists who are big supporters of Retin-A, the answer is settled: starting Retin-A when you are younger is better for your skin.

What Type of Retin-A to Use

When you book your appointment with your dermatologist to get your prescription of Retin-A, can you feel confident that your doctor will discuss with you all the potential outcomes and the strengths of the different prescriptions available? It all depends on your dermatologist. Regardless of your dermatologist's professional ability, you will still want all the information necessary so you can be a good consumer and a knowledgeable patient.

There are several concentrations of Retin-A available. In descending order of strength, starting with the most potent, they are 0.05 percent liquid, 0.025 percent gel, 0.01 percent gel, 0.1 percent cream, 0.05 percent cream, and 0.025 percent cream. Generally speaking, for those getting a prescription of Retin-A for sun-damaged skin, the initial choice is usually the 0.025 percent cream. This is considered to be the most gentle of all the formulations. It is almost always the beginning step when using Retin-A because it provides the least amount of irritation to the face. But it is not the final step. The stronger dose—at least the 0.05 percent cream and eventually the 0.1 percent cream—are the most desirable because they will have the biggest effect on sun-damaged skin. The reason to start with the weakest strength and work your way up is so your skin can adjust slowly to the effects of Retin-A, minimizing the irritation and dryness.

There are vast differences between the gel and liquid Retin-A and the cream Retin-A. The gel and liquid are much more potent than any of the creams, and they can cause a greater degree of dryness and irritation. It is never recommended that anyone with sun-damaged skin use the gel or liquid formulas.

There is a difference between the type of Retin-A prescribed for sun-damaged skin versus skin that breaks out. Ordinarily, when Retin-A is being prescribed for acned skin, the gel or liquid strengths are given. The assumption is that acned skin can handle the irritation and dryness caused by using a stronger form of Retin-A. I do not agree with that thinking at all. I believe that all skin types are better off with the cream version to start with. There is no distinction between the degree of irritation or dryness someone with acne will experience versus that which someone with sun-damaged skin will experience. Irritation and dryness can be severe and painful regardless of skin type. I've interviewed a number of people who were using the Retin-A gel for their acne and were also using a moisturizer to minimize the irritation and dryness. They would have been better off minimizing the irritation to begin with by using the cream version of Retin-A. The cream is less potent than the gel, which would help lessen the initial side effects of Retin-A. Plus, the gel and liquid Retin-A contain alcohol, which can increase irritation and dryness measurably.

The other reason using the gel or liquid is usually recommended for acned skin types is that the effects of Retin-A increase in an alcohol base as opposed to a cream base. In those cases where the additional strength is necessary, it would still be preferable to start slowly, step by step, adapting the skin to the onslaught of the stronger prescriptions by starting with the less potent creams and working up.

I mentioned before that the 0.025 percent cream was only the first step in using Retin-A. The idea is not to stay with the 0.025 percent cream indefinitely, but to move on to the stronger 0.05 percent cream as the skin adjusts to the weaker dose and the irritation and dryness subside. Unfortunately, there is every chance that the irritation and dryness will return when you change to the higher strength, but the irritation and dryness at both levels will not be as great as if you had used the 0.05 percent right from the very start. Dr. Kligman feels it should be everyone's goal to get to the point where they are using the strong 0.1 percent cream. The stronger the Retin-A, the better it works.

Before You Start

If you are going to be successful using Retin-A, there are a few things you need to know about cleansing your face in order to minimize the inherent irritation and dryness that come from using it. One week before you start Retin-A, *stop* using all irritating skin care products on the face. Adhering to the following warnings will help you survive treatment with reduced discomfort and difficulty.

Do not use any creams that contain fragrance or coloring agents.
Do not wipe makeup off your face; the wiping will irritate the skin.
Do not use any astringents, toners, or fresheners whatsoever that contain any irritants.
Do not use three percent hydrogen peroxide solution.
Do not use any facial masks of any kind.
Do not use any over-the-counter products designed for acned or oily skin.
Do not use bar soaps of any kind on the face.
Do not use washcloths, or scrubbing or buffing products on the face.
Do not dry your face by rubbing it with a towel; dab only.
Do not sit in a dry or steam sauna.
Do not get a facial or facial massage. Even the gentlest rubbing can prove to be too irritating for someone starting to use Retin-A.

Do not go outside without sunscreen protection.
Do not rub or touch your face more than necessary.
Do not use any products that contain irritating ingredients.
Do not use hot water directly on the face.

Now that you know what not to do, it is equally important for you to know exactly what to do. This list is shorter but just as essential in the first few months of application.

Do be as gentle as possible with your skin.
Do clean your face with Cetaphil Lotion or a water-soluble cleanser that doesn't contain fragrance, coloring agents, or irritating cleansing agents.
Do use tepid water only.
Do use a moisturizer that does not contain fragrance, coloring agents, or irritants.
Do use a sunscreen with an SPF of 15 or greater during the day.
Do be patient; the results happen slowly over a period of time.

If you are breaking out or have oily skin, you will want to use the baking soda judiciously or not at all depending on how dry and irritated your skin becomes. This "do" list is as important as the "do not" list. Both will save your face and make using Retin-A relatively easy.

After You Start

People often make mistakes applying Retin-A in the beginning. The most frequent errors are: using too much, applying it too often, applying it with cotton balls or swabs, and applying it only over wrinkles. All of these mistakes will make using Retin-A either more problematic or more displeasing than it need be.

The way to apply Retin-A is with your fingertips. It won't hurt your fingers unless you have eczema or psoriasis, in which case you would want to discuss that with your doctor. Use a small amount and spread it evenly all over the face. In most cases, a small tube will last at least two months. Overusing Retin-A will increase the chance that you will develop inflammation and swelling. Cotton balls or swabs will absorb most of the Retin-A and waste your money. You will get a much more even spread if you use your fingers.

Be sure to use the Retin-A all over your face, and do not concentrate only on the wrinkles. There is no proof that the Retin-A will get rid of wrinkles, and yet there is every reason to believe that the entire face will benefit from the effect of increased cell turnover and color improvement. Speaking of application, do not forget the skin around the eye area. The eye area is just as sun-damaged as the rest of the face, so you might as well use it there and get all the benefits possible. (Check with your dermatologist to be sure he agrees with Retin-A usage in the eye area.) By the way, if you do use Retin-A on the very delicate skin around the eye, consider diluting a small amount of the cream with an equal portion of Cetaphil Lotion before applying it. Again, see if your dermatologist agrees with this method. Do not expect to see a big change in the bags or sagging skin around the eye. The improvement will mostly be in texture and skin color; you're not getting a face-lift.

The other thing that is important to remember when using Retin-A is to follow your doctor's instructions. Basically, the suggested routine is to apply Retin-A at night only, after the face is washed. Most dermatologists suggest waiting twenty minutes after you wash the face before applying the Retin-A. The reason for this is to be sure that there is no alkali detergent residue left on the face, which could negate the effect of acid-based Retin-A. If you use the Cetaphil Lotion, there would be no need to wait because there is no alkali detergent in Cetaphil. For the most part, when it comes to other cleansers, particularly soap, you will want to wait the twenty minutes before applying the Retin-A.

Once you start using Retin-A, expect irritation and dryness to develop within the first week of usage. The skin may begin to peel, develop dry, scaly patches, and possibly burn and itch. If you find that these side effects are more than your skin can comfortably handle, you may want to cut back your frequency of use. In the beginning you can avoid some of the irritation by applying the Retin-A only two or three times a week instead of every day, and this would slowly build up your skin's tolerance. If your skin is still too irritated, then try mixing half your nightly application of Retin-A with an equal amount of the Cetaphil Lotion before applying it to the face. Those two steps, reducing the frequency of application and cutting the normal amount you use in half with the Cetaphil Lotion, can reduce the skin's severe reaction to Retin-A.

Another option for dealing with severe irritation and dry patches is to use a topical cortisone cream. You can either get a prescription for one from your doctor, or you can try a nonprescription hydrocortisone cream. Use either type of cortisone cream in the morning, after you wash your face with the Cetaphil Lotion but before you put on your moisturizer with sunscreen. If your skin becomes very dry, your moisturizer can be reapplied several times a day as needed. Between using the Cetaphil Lotion as your cleanser twice a day, a moisturizing sunscreen during the day, and a topical cortisone cream as needed, you should be able to alleviate most of the side effects as they show up.

You will be pleased to know that most of the irritation should stop after a few weeks—in extreme situations after a few months—depending on your skin's sensitivity. Your skin wants to do what the Retin-A is helping it do, so it is only a matter of time before the skin adapts to the treatment.

Warning: *Retin-A can make the face sun-sensitive. That doesn't mean you can't go outside or play in the sun; it just means that you need to be meticulous about applying a strong sunscreen to protect the face. Retin-A keeps the skin in a constant state of peeling, leaving the surface layer more vulnerable then usual to the rays of the sun. Be aware of this and act accordingly. It never hurts to get your doctor's feedback before you do anything. An SPF of 15 or greater would be preferred. If you think you can tan and still use Retin-A to prevent the effects of sun exposure, think again. Any amount of tanning you do while using Retin-A not only negates the effectiveness of using it, but can also be dangerous for the skin.*

If you do everything according to plan, the treatment procedure for Retin-A on sun-damaged skin should show noticeable results in about three to four months. Again, to assure the path to success is paved with gold, be certain you are starting with a low concentration of Retin-A—the 0.025 percent cream is preferred—to see how your skin will react. The suggested application is to use the Retin-A at night all by itself without a moisturizer, but if your skin requires a moisturizer to feel comfortable, don't hesitate to use one. In the morning, after cleansing the face, apply a moisturizer with a sunscreen of SPF 15 or greater as needed. Again, if irritation shows up, you can change from using the Retin-A every night to every other night or mix half the amount you would normally use with an equal amount of the Cetaphil Lotion at night, and in the morning apply a cortisone cream over the irritated areas. Always be sure to check with your dermatologist first before modifying your treatment.

What About Wearing Makeup?

Good question, but I'm not so sure you're going to like the answer. For the first several weeks you will probably find it best not to wear much makeup at all, particularly foundation. Personally, I found that my flaking and peeling skin looked worse when I wore foundation. Eyeshadows and blushes will also go on choppy over dry, irritated skin. Wearing moisturizer might help, but it still may look like there's rough skin under there. For the first month or two you should have no problem wearing mascara, lipstick, and eyeliner. For me, after six weeks of using Retin-A my makeup did start to go on smoother, but there were still some dry patches that looked more dry and flaky with makeup on, especially under the eyes. This is one territory you will have to test for yourself. The one thing you will definitely need to change is your foundation if you normally wear an oil-free foundation that goes on rather dry; you will want to switch to a water-based foundation that contains a small amount of oil. Do not use any foundations that contain alcohol or glycerin (large amounts of glycerin can cause skin to become irritated). Everything else should be able to stay the same.

How Long Do I Have to Use the Retin-A?

According to Dr. Kligman, you can start using Retin-A and a strong sunscreen as soon as you want to and for as long as you want to. His feelings are that, because of what Retin-A can do for the skin, you can be on it for the rest of your life if you are so inclined—particularly if you want to continue seeing results. After about a year of regular nightly applications of the strongest percentage of Retin-A your doctor prescribes, Dr. Kligman feels a maintenance program of regular intermittent use can be continued indefinitely. Dr. Kligman suggests that after you have used Retin-A regularly for a year or more you should stop using it for three to four months and then start again using it on a daily (nightly) basis. Then for the rest of your life you can alternate three to four months on and three to four months off.

Dr. Kligman warns that entirely discontinuing use can return the skin to its original condition. Skin seems to be preprogrammed to respond to sun damage and decrease in cell production as we age. In the long run, what you choose to do is up to you and your doctor.

Step by Step—What to Do on Retin-A Therapy

1 One to two weeks before you begin applying Retin-A, stop using all forms of soap, alcohol-based products, washcloths, and scrub products—including baking soda, moisturizers that contain fragrance or coloring agents, facial treatments for acne, facial masks including milk of magnesia, extended periods of time in dry or steam saunas, facials, and cosmetics that contain irritating ingredients.

2 Twice a day wash your face with Cetaphil Lotion. Use the Cetaphil Lotion to remove your makeup. Do not wipe off makeup since the wiping can prove to be very irritating to the skin. If you break out, massage very gently with baking soda only the blemishes that rudely show up. Do not massage the baking soda anywhere else.

3 At night, twenty minutes after you've washed and dabbed your skin dry, apply a small amount of the 0.025 percent Retin-A cream over the entire face, including the area under the eye and on the eyelid. Do not use your moisturizer at night.

4 In the morning, after you've washed your face with Cetaphil Lotion, apply a moisturizer that contains a sunscreen of SPF 15 or greater.

5 By the third or fourth day you may notice dryness and dry patches. Your face may also feel unusually sensitive and slightly itchy. The sides of your nose and the sides of your mouth may be cracked and dry. You may want to avoid applying the Retin-A to these areas on a daily basis and apply it only every other day. The irritation will eventually go away, but it is something that must be tolerated in the beginning.

6 If the irritation and dryness are causing you problems, you may want to cut down your application of Retin-A to every other night or to three times a week. Another option is to dilute your nightly application by mixing half of what you would normally use with the Cetaphil Lotion and then applying that mixture to the face. (Cetaphil Lotion is so gentle it is okay to leave it on the face overnight.) Keep in mind, though, that it is preferable to apply Retin-A in full strength every night in order to see the desired results sooner.

7 Another way to combat the irritation is to apply a cortisone cream, either prescription or nonprescription, in the morning to those extremely aggravated areas on your face that are driving you crazy. (Using the cortisone cream is only a temporary remedy and should not be done on a regular basis. Regular use of cortisone creams, particularly prescription cortisone creams, can damage the skin and cause wrinkles.)

8 If it is absolutely necessary for you to alleviate some of the discomfort from the dryness at night, try using your favorite moisturizer at least thirty minutes after you've applied the Retin-A. Be sure to find out if your doctor agrees with this step.

9 If you are not experiencing any irritation or dryness after the first few weeks of using the 0.025 percent cream, you will want to move on to the 0.05 percent cream at this time. The same is true for those who start with the 0.05 percent cream and do not experience any irritation. You will want to move on to the 0.1 percent cream.

10 You can apply makeup as you normally would. The only exception to that would be if you were using a foundation base that contained alcohol or was specifically labeled as being oil-free. When using Retin-A, the only way you will find relief from dryness is to supply the skin with a little bit of oil. For some women, a foundation can make the skin look even more dehydrated and flaky than it is. Not wearing a foundation for a few weeks or until the dryness subsides may be the best thing to do.

11 Try not to scratch or rub the skin no matter how much it itches.

12 If you have any questions, consult your dermatologist. There is also a consumer hot line provided by the Ortho division of Johnson & Johnson (the people who make Retin-A). You can call them at (800) 526–3967. Be aware when you call that you may be encouraged to use Johnson & Johnson's products in conjunction with Retin-A (such as Purpose soap and Purpose moisturizer, which you can ignore, or Sundown sunscreens, which are an option), but they will also have answers to other practical questions that involve use rather than skin care.

What Happened to Me

I included this section in the last edition of *Blue Eyeshadow Should Still Be Illegal*. It is the only section of the book that has required no revision. I feel that it is a good documentation of what can happen when you first encounter Retin-A. You may have different experiences, but judging from the women I've interviewed, what I went through, to one extent or another, was fairly normal. The only thing I am adding to this section is what happened to me over the three years after I published the second edition of this book. That part of my relationship with Retin-A also seems to be fairly normal. As of this writing I have been using Retin-A on and off for a total of three years.

Day 1. I spent $30 for a rather large tube of Retin-A in a 0.05 percent cream base. I was told this would be about a three- to four-month supply. I have been very good about not using the baking soda all over my face. I only used the baking soda and three percent hydrogen peroxide solution on blemishes. I also purchased a $15 tube of cortisone cream that was safe to use on the face. I applied the Retin-A as directed, being extra careful to get it right next to my lashes, and then went to bed. The first night went by relatively uneventfully.

Day 2. Excitedly I called my friend Julie to tell her that nothing had happened but I was looking forward with excitement to the next few weeks. The second night went pretty much like the first.

Day 3. I woke up with a tiny rash on my forehead. I also had several blemishes on my chin and cheek. My skin had a noticeable pinkness to it, as if I had been out in the sun for an hour or so without a sunscreen. I also felt a tingling sensation all over my face. After I washed my face with Cetaphil Lotion, I massaged the blemishes with baking soda. When my face was rinsed and dried I applied the cortisone cream to the rash on my forehead. That night I applied the Retin-A as I had before and went to bed.

Day 6. Wow, did my eyes itch, and the sides of my lips were cracked and dry. Actually, my whole face felt slightly itchy. The blemishes and rash on my forehead had disappeared so I stopped using the baking soda and three percent hydrogen peroxide solution altogether. I'd used the cortisone cream over the sides of my nose and at the corners of my mouth again for the second night in a row. There was a slight amount of dryness on my cheeks but nothing to complain about. Because I have naturally oily skin and a tendency to break out, I still had not found it necessary to use a moisturizer, but I had one ready just in case. Before I went to bed I put on the Retin-A, trying to keep my hands off my itchy face.

Day 10. The irritation did not seem to be so bad that morning, although the sides of my lips were still dry and cracked and my eyes still felt itchy. There was also flaky dry skin all over my face. My husband had started staring closely at my face, saying, "You're paying someone to do this to your skin?" I hoped that at the end of the month we both would notice a difference. I've decided to be patient and see the thing through, at least until the end of the tube.

Day 14. I called Julie again to tell her that my face was feeling much less irritated and itchy, my eyes weren't driving me crazy, the peeling on my cheeks had calmed down, and the cracks on the sides of my lips were better, too. I had only been applying the cortisone cream every other day to the sides of my nose and the corners of my lips. I had used the baking soda two or three times, in the morning only, very gently all over my face to help remove some of the scaling, but that was it. I hadn't had any blemishes to speak of and my face had a nice pinkness all over. All in all, I was remaining skeptical. I wasn't going to get my hopes up; I was just going to enjoy my skin's semi-return to normality and see if it lasted.

Day 16. Today Julie called me. She wanted to know how things were going. She also said most of her friends were curious, too. I reported in and said I was pleased with what was happening to my face but still apprehensive. I told her that I was noticing a change in the few whiteheads I have that never seem to go away—those small, hard white lumps that don't do anything on the face but sit there seemed to be breaking up. If they really did dissolve and go away, that would be wonderful.

Day 18. My skin was definitely doing better. My forehead was still a little itchy, but I put some cortisone cream on and was sure it would go away quickly. My eyes hardly itched at all and the sides of my lips weren't cracked anymore. I had stopped applying cortisone cream to those areas a few days ago. My skin felt a little tight and there was some dryness, but it wasn't bad. I was concerned about what would happen to my acne when my menstrual cycle showed up in the next few days, but I hoped for the best. Later that day a friend called to tell me that her hairdresser had said that there had been reports of Retin-A causing some people to bleed right through their skin! I asked where the hairdresser had heard that; she said he'd heard it from a client who'd heard it from a friend. I said he should stick to cutting hair and stay away from medical assessments. Retin-A, in the twenty-five years that it had been used as an acne treatment, had never produced such an effect. Nor had any other research documented such absurdity. If the skin became that irritated, like the sides of my mouth had, perhaps a little bleeding would occur from the cracked skin. In that case, all that would be needed would be to stop the Retin-A or to apply a cortisone cream to the irritated areas. (As I explained before, if irritation is severe you need to cut back your frequency of application or dilute the application with Cetaphil Lotion. There are a lot of things you can do to reduce the irritation, way before any serious trouble sets in.)

Day 20. Except for a general sensation of tenderness all over my face and a bit of dryness on my cheeks, everything seemed to be back to normal. Some of those whiteheads I'd been hoping would go away were less noticeable but still there. There was no difference in the lines on my face, but then again, I didn't have many lines anyway. I still seemed to have my share of blemishes, which I dealt with as they popped up.

Day 24. My period started and everything seemed fairly normal. I still had my usual share of menstrual acne, but nothing a little baking soda and three percent hydrogen peroxide solution couldn't handle. My eyes had been a little more sensitive than normal, but it wasn't that uncomfortable.

Day 31. The sides of my lips became dry again, so I used the cortisone cream to help alleviate the irritation. My forehead seemed to be more sensitive to the Retin-A than any other part of my face. I didn't want to overuse the cortisone cream, so I cut back the Retin-A application on my forehead to every other night.

Day 40. I was surprised at how good my face felt. Other than the routine of applying Retin-A every night and using the baking soda only when I needed it, everything seemed to be as it should be. I did notice a difference in the surface texture of my skin; it felt smoother, and even where I was breaking out it felt somewhat softer.

Day 43. I went to bed late and forgot to use the Retin-A. I guess I'm becoming more relaxed about the whole experience.

Day 47. It was warm in Seattle and I went for a bike ride with my husband, being sure to apply a strong sunscreen before we went. I also packed the sunscreen with me in case we were gone for more than two hours so I could reapply the sunscreen to maintain protection.

Day 49. My skin started flaking like crazy. It could be that the little bit of sun exposure I got the other day affected my skin. I gently used the baking soda all over my face and it seemed to take care of it. By the way, a few days ago I stopped using the Retin-A on my forehead altogether. I still seemed to get a rash every time I used it, and I wasn't willing to continue reapplying the cortisone cream that frequently. Cortisone creams, with constant use, can negate the positive effects of the Retin-A and damage the skin.

Day 55. I'd been a little lazier than usual and skipped a couple of nights. I put the Retin-A on in the morning instead and everything seemed to go smoothly. I found that my face was much less sensitive than it had been when I started the whole process. Unfortunately, my face still had its share of blemishes. So much for Retin-A being an acne medication as far as my face is concerned.

Day 72. I'd been more routine about using Retin-A every night or in the morning. I started using it on my forehead again with no problems at all. After almost three months of using Retin-A, I've learned that it is indeed an experience. I have decided to continue regular daily applications for the next nine months and will probably continue with a maintenance program of twice a week after that. Unless the medical journals report otherwise, I'm convinced that Retin-A is beneficial for the skin. My face feels smoother and, to a lesser degree, looks it, too. Not a startling change, but enough to keep me interested.

End of second year. I found that I had a problem being disciplined about using the Retin-A every night. When I did use it on a regular basis, I liked the way my skin felt; the texture and color were really much better, but my wrinkles were still here and there were even some new ones. I would like to be more committed to the routine, but that wasn't easy for me. I tried to keep it up, and I needed to reschedule an appointment with my dermatologist. That in itself seemed to be difficult to organize.

End of third year. Same as the second year, except I was off Retin-A more than I was on it. Being committed to using this cream is difficult—I wish it wasn't. I do like the way my skin looks and feels when I use it, but the regular application is difficult to keep up. Then, after I let six months lapse without using Retin-A, I didn't want to go through getting used to it again. What a dilemma! For now I am still off it, but I earnestly want to start again. I'll let you know what happens in future updates.

Questions and Answers— Clearing the Rumors

Q. Is it true, what I've heard, that not all women can use Retin-A?

A. That is true, but for only a very small percentage of the population. Someone with severe dermatitis or some other traumatic skin malady or extreme skin sensitivity should probably avoid using it. But in those situations the dermatologist would be the one to determine the advantages and disadvantages of Retin-A therapy. Otherwise, Retin-A has such minor side effects that, despite being uncomfortable, it is essentially harmless to use.

Q. Is the irritation caused by Retin-A so bad that it actually hurts the skin, as I've read?

A. I'm not sure what you've read or what you mean by the term *hurts the skin*. Some people will react more severely than others to Retin-A therapy, and in those cases it would be best to stop using it and consult your dermatologist. But if you mean, *Does it permanently hurt the skin?*—that is not likely. In the twenty-five years or so that Retin-A has been used as a prescription drug for acne, no permanent damage has been documented. The discomfort that is caused by the irritating side effects of Retin-A will eventually stop with continued applications—in a few weeks to a few months, depending on your skin's sensitivities.

Q. When I've used Retin-A in the past my doctor told me to continue using the skin care routine I had already been using. Do you think that's a good idea?

A. Depending on the skin care routine, I think it can be a great idea or a totally rotten one. If you are washing your face twice a day with Cetaphil Lotion or some other nonfragranced, nonirritating, soap-free cleanser, massaging occasional blemishes with a little baking soda, and using a moisturizing sunscreen with an SPF of 15 or greater, that would be perfect. But if you're using scrub products, astringents or toners that contain irritating ingredients, washcloths, soaps, fragranced moisturizers, facial masks, or you're steaming your face, your skin may overreact to

Retin-A. Much of the irritation can be avoided if you are as absolutely gentle as possible when cleansing your face.

Q. I received a tube of Retin-A from a friend. Is it safe to use it without seeing a doctor first?

A. It is probably safe but not very smart. Retin-A truly has few to no serious side effects that would not be eliminated if you simply stopped using it. What isn't smart, especially if you want to achieve positive results, is to forgo having your skin's reaction to the Retin-A monitored. If your skin reacts severely to the treatment, you can quickly get a prescription for a cortisone cream to reduce the initial irritation that accompanies the first applications. The other problem is that Retin-A comes in a few different strengths and bases. You will want to be sure you are using the one that is least likely to cause irritation and then move on to the stronger strengths when it is appropriate to do so. And finally, Retin-A is a drug, and because all skins are different, it wouldn't hurt to check yours out with a doctor before you begin treatment.

Q. How old do I have to be before I start using Retin-A?

A. That depends on what you want and how sun-damaged your skin is. Retin-A performs a number of functions that have benefits for all people who go out in the sun or are in the process of growing up. Basically the time to start is when you notice that your skin is showing signs of sun damage, and that can develop in your early twenties. The typical age for women to start using Retin-A is between thirty and forty-five. But if you want to prevent problems from sun-damaged skin you can never start too young to wear a sunscreen and use Retin-A. Remember, once you use Retin-A on a regular basis for a year, you do not have to continue daily usage. After the first year you could go on a maintenance program that can be handled a couple of ways: you could cut your applications to three times a week or you could use the Retin-A for three to four months, stop for three to four months, and then start again.

Q. I've heard that Retin-A is expensive. Is it?

A. Whether or not something is perceived as expensive is always a relative question. What seems overpriced to you may not be for me and vice versa. In my opinion Retin-A couldn't be cheaper. The cost can vary, but it averages out to around $30 for a large tube that should last you three to four and possibly up to six months.

Q. What about wearing makeup?

A. Makeup should be no problem, unless, of course, your face is reacting severely to the Retin-A or peeling excessively. There are no inherent complications in wearing makeup, assuming that the foundation you're using doesn't contain alcohol or any other drying ingredients. If your face is going through a phase of irritation and dryness, and you haven't found any relief from the cortisone cream or your moisturizer, you will have problems wearing makeup comfortably. This period of skin sensitivity should end soon. In the meantime, you may want to consider wearing only a moisturizer with sunscreen on your face during the day along with mascara, eyeliner, and lipstick. Your face will let you know when you can start putting foundation and blush on again smoothly.

Q. Is Retin-A really an anti-wrinkle cream?

A. The safest and most accurate answer to your question, as far as I know, is that Retin-A is probably an effective anti-effects-of-sun-damaged-skin cream and an anti-cell-aging cream. What Retin-A does for the skin is to change and improve some of the damage that happens to the skin from sitting in the sun. Will that visibly change your wrinkles? Probably not. What it will do is change the surface appearance of your skin to that of a more healthy, pre-sun-damaged condition.

Q. If I don't sit in the sun, will Retin-A make a difference on my skin?

A. Sitting in the sun is only one way your skin gets hit by the sun. Walking outside is another. For those of us who drive to work or spend time in the park, our faces are exposed to the sun enough that using Retin-A could make a positive difference.

Q. I haven't been a sun worshipper since I was twenty-five. Won't that prevent my skin from developing sun damage?

A. It's good that you've stopped exposing your face to the damaging rays of the sun because that will prevent further damage, but it won't change the damage that was done when you were younger. Most of the damage to your skin was done years ago.

Chapter Four
Cosmetic Surgery—The Art of Cutting Away Wrinkles

Filling in the Lines

After telling you that moisturizers, wrinkle creams, facials, and facial exercises can't change one wrinkle on your face, I should give you some information about what *can* have a dramatic effect on wrinkles. The only options for significantly erasing wrinkles on a long-term basis are available from cosmetics surgeons and dermatologists. (When I talk about *dramatic change* in the appearance of wrinkles, please note that I am not referring to Retin-A. *Dramatic change* refers to any procedure that would remove most wrinkles from your face for a period of years. Retin-A does not produce dramatic results when it comes to changing wrinkles. Retin-A's effects on wrinkles, particularly deep wrinkles, are regarded as being very subtle to imperceptible.)

The cosmetic surgeries and procedures that are available to anyone who wants to and can afford to permanently or semipermanently change their appearance are mind-boggling. Some of the procedures are simple, and some of them seem miraculous. Whether it be straightening a nose or plumping up a sagging laugh line or a major reconstructive effort such as setting an accident victim's cranial structure back to normal, there are things happening in the world of cosmetic medicine you might not have given a passing thought to just a few years ago.

Nose jobs, chin implants, cheek implants, eye tucks, orthodontics, teeth bonding, jaw restructuring, teeth restructuring, collagen injections, face-lifts, breast implants, breast reductions, liposuction, tummy tucks, and buttock tucks are some of the more common medical cosmetic procedures you've probably read or heard about. As you already may know, each one of these options can be done solo or in tandem with one or more of the others. When you consider the endless possible combinations, you can see that in the hands of the right team of experts, almost any look, within reason, can be attempted and perhaps realized.

Before I start sounding too much like an ad for cosmetic surgery, let me quickly put the above elaboration into perspective. I am not encouraging everyone to run out and get their bottom lifted or their eyes tucked. What I'm doing is sharing my astonishment at what is happening out there in the arena of cosmetic surgery. I did not intend this book to be a complete reference guide for those of you who need detailed consumer-oriented information about a specific cosmetic surgery. But I am including several sections on the subject so you can begin to formulate in your mind what the emotional ramifications of cosmetic surgery can be and what you can do once you make your decision.

To Lift or Not to Lift

What woman crossing the threshold of mid-life into her forties hasn't calculated what impact a face-lift, eye tuck, collagen injection, or chemical face peel might have on her face? How many of us have pulled at our faces to adjust the skin more tightly around our chin or eyes to see what it would look like if a little skin were snipped here or cut there? And how many of us have discussed with envy or disdain what any one of a number of celebrities looked like after they had their faces or bodies readjusted?

For many people in the United States, the final solution to aging is the cosmetic surgeon, and as a result of this belief, the statistics on cosmetic surgery are nothing less than astounding. I personally am amazed at the number of women I know who have had face-lifts, eye tucks, and nose reductions in just the past year or two.

The entire subject of cosmetic surgery poses more questions than meet the eye. The typical queries cover what types of procedures are available and what the probable results are, both negative and positive, that can be expected of medical anti-aging solutions. Although these questions are essential to explore and understand, they are not necessarily the first ones to ask. The more difficult questions to ponder are the ones we should be most concerned about—those that have nothing to do with technicalities. The questions we need to ask ourselves are, Why do we want to do all this stuff to ourselves? Why can't we just be fine the way we are? What do we hope to gain from looking unwrinkled and unsagged?

It's a provocative notion to examine why so many of us want to cut, inject, or rub away parts of our bodies that are neither dangerous to our health nor lethal. It could be explained simply by repeating the standard one-liner, "If people want to look better or younger, and modern medicine can provide that vehicle, why not?" Asking "why not" begs the question.

That answer is not only simplistic, it encourages us to avoid looking at the emotional aspect these surgeries can have on the individual. If we stop and look inside ourselves, and contemplate what it means to leave youth behind, our emotions may run the entire gamut from fear to relief, but probably not to joy. For each of us who has ever wondered what our face would be like minus a sag or a line here and there has looked indirectly at our society's most socially acceptable fear: growing older.

There are many philosophical, sociological, and psychological issues that affect our decision to have cosmetic surgery, particularly face-lifts and eye tucks. Sociologically, we live a lot longer than we did a mere seventy-five years ago, which means we have a lot more aging to put up with than ever before. Philosophically, I earnestly believe that all of us are inherently fine just the way we are, but I am also aware that we live in a society that puts a great emphasis on personal appearance. Many studies demonstrate that the better you look, the healthier you are, the more successful you can be, and the greater the chances are that you will receive preferential treatment wherever you go. And finally, when it comes to our own psychological well-being, I'm all too aware of the emotional pain caused by living in a world that is overwhelmingly preoccupied with surface appearance while de-emphasizing the importance of being worthwhile human beings. Sometimes, it seems easier to ignore the more profound issues and just schedule an appointment with the best cosmetic surgeon we can find. In the long run, most women I interviewed would rather cut five to ten years from their appearance than stare at their departing youth every day.

Regrettably, I have no specific suggestions that can point the way through the personal and social dilemmas of deciding whether or not a particular cosmetic surgery or procedure is indeed the best thing for you emotionally. But I encourage you to consider not only the information that follows but also the larger social issues before making *your* final decision.

Let me stress one point: my suggestions about looking inside ourselves first for our reasons for wanting to get a face-lift or other procedure does not mean I am against cosmetic surgery. I have seen the extraordinary results of these surgeries and would consider cosmetic surgery for myself. I also believe that there is nothing inherently vain or narcissistic about wanting to look younger via cosmetic surgery. Nor is cosmetic surgery an admission of failure or a proof of old age. It's your right to want to look younger and more attractive; that may be considered vain in some cultures, but in the United States, it is socially acceptable.

Still, I am worried about the startling increase in cosmetic surgeries being performed in this country. I see it as an indicator of how we overlook the special beauty that comes with growing up. Unless we face up to who we are as women over forty, fifty, sixty, or seventy and begin to celebrate those changes, we are destined to eventually catch up with our worst fear. No matter how many wrinkles we can cut away, we still have to deal with what it means to not be young anymore. The risk we take by not dealing with this fact, besides never enjoying the age we are, is that of looking like an overtight caricature of a female. If you have seen women who have had more than one face-lift or just one bad face-lift, you know what I'm talking about.

If we believe that cosmetic surgery can imbue us with some type of instant happiness or self-esteem, we are only fooling ourselves. Collagen injections and face-lifts cause skin-deep physical changes. The energy and internal peace needed for enjoying life and finding happiness can't be stitched into a face, nor can the perplexities of day-to-day stress be smoothed away by filling in wrinkles. As hackneyed as this may sound, it bears repeating because it is the absolute truth: joy and happiness are not purchasable commodities. The passion for living a wonderful existence comes from within, and only you can make that a reality.

I do not intend to scare you away from cosmetic surgery—just the opposite. Hopefully it will make you stronger in your resolve and belief in yourself. The next step, then, is reviewing the practical, graphic information about cosmetic surgery that you still need to know. I encourage you to do all your homework before you embark on a trip to a cosmetic surgeon's office. There are many things that can go wrong with any surgery, and cosmetic surgery is no exception. I am often shocked by the number of women who decide to go ahead with a particular cosmetic surgery having no more information than the recommendation of a friend of a friend who received a good face-lift from Dr. So-and-So. There are crucial factors, both positive and negative, that you must know about before you decide to go ahead with any specific type of cosmetic surgery. Once you have researched your risks, you must choose which cosmetic surgeon you will trust with your face or body and what questions to ask him or her.

When Should You Have Cosmetic Surgery?

This is a controversial question. Many cosmetic surgeons say that the best age is within five years from the time you first start thinking about it. The basic concept is that the younger you are when you have the surgery, the better the outcome will be. It seems that those men and women who have cosmetic surgery done before the age of fifty-five experience better results and longer-lasting effects than older people. The farther the skin sags and wrinkles, the harder it is to snip and tuck it back into shape without overpulling and destroying natural facial contours. There is, however, a fine line between having cosmetic surgery too young versus having it too old. If there is not enough sagging, there is little benefit to be realized, and the success of the surgery is minimized. Perhaps the best determining factors should be your desire to have it done and the opinion of at least two qualified surgeons that the potential results warrant the surgery.

The other reason to have cosmetic surgery now as opposed to later is that you will reap the rewards that much sooner. If you are concerned about the aging of your face and know that you will eventually jump in and have cosmetic surgery, then waiting is an emotional game you play with yourself to no one's advantage. Perhaps you are under the assumption that being old and shriveled is the main reason someone should consider cosmetic surgery. That is not the case. Cosmetic surgery is done mainly for the purpose of beauty, and beauty alone, and it should have nothing to do with age. Being more beautiful physically in and of itself is a very good reason to consider cosmetic surgery.

If you decide to have cosmetic surgery, don't do it because some friend has suggested it or recommended a doctor. Consider it over a period of time and back up your thinking with research and consultations with more than one physician. This is not a haircut; this is surgery. "Jump on in, the water is fine" is not sound advice when you are electing to have any surgery.

The Mastery of the Face-Lift

The surgical skill and knowledge required to perform the perfect face-lift is astounding. This is no small task. The demand for cosmetic surgery in general is increasing at a phenomenal rate, mostly because the population—particularly the baby boomers, who are now well into their forties—is not happy losing its youth. The more the demand increases, the more cosmetic surgeons are needed. The number of cosmetic surgeons graduating into practices of their own can barely keep up with the rising demand for their services.

What does all that mean for the consumer? That there are a lot of cosmetic surgeons out there and that finding the best-trained one is more essential than ever.

What is the difference between a qualified surgeon and a surgeon who is not only qualified but an artist? The major distinctions are in the attention to detail during surgery and the knowledge of what can happen after the surgery is over. Adroit surgeons will not only lift the sagging skin and wrinkles from the face, they will also attend to such nuances as lifting drooping eyebrows or shortening sinking earlobes. The ingenious cosmetic surgeon will know how to place scars so they are well hidden behind ears or hairlines. How an incision is made and how a scar is placed is integral to the quality of the lift. For example, along the lower eye, a well-placed incision—that does not damage the muscle—can create a scar that will not pull downward during the healing process and cause the scar to protrude. One well-known surgeon places an incision in the crease of the neck for some of his face-lift patients. The purpose of his technique is to reduce the difficult-to-remove lines that run from the corners of the nose to the mouth. Placing the scar along the fold of the neck supposedly better hides an otherwise obvious scar that is usually placed next to the ear. Another surgeon is acclaimed for her ability to eliminate the surprised look typically associated with overpulled face-lifts. How can you determine whether your surgeon is accomplished in all these various techniques? That is the next step.

How to Shop for a Cosmetic Surgeon

This is not an easy task. In general, most Americans are not good consumers when it comes to the entire world of medicine. We tend to stick with whomever was recommended by someone we know or the last medical professional we talked to. The same is true for the way we deal with finding a cosmetic surgeon. Once we've scheduled an appointment, it doesn't seem to matter how the doctor treats us, how much time is spent with us before surgery and after, how much experience the doctor has, how many satisfied patients were offered as referrals, or what medical boards the doctor belongs to. Yet all these are integral pieces of information you need to make a decision about any doctor you give your body or face to for care. Almost all of the twenty-five women I interviewed who had undergone some type of cosmetic surgery did not pose any of these questions to their surgeons, nor did they seem to think it was important. They all had chosen the doctor who performed their surgeries because they had been recommended by a friend or a friend of a friend. That is not the best way to choose a cosmetic surgeon. The result of one surgery does not tell you much. It can be a good place to start, but it should not be the definitive criterion.

It isn't easy being a good consumer in this arena, but believe me, the differences that exist out there among surgeons are vast. I'm not just talking about the differences between a doctor who does a bad face-lift and a doctor who does a good one, although that is critical. I'm talking about the difference between a doctor who does a good face-lift and a doctor who can do a great one.

The best place to start when shopping for a cosmetic surgeon is to call the nearest medical teaching facility, ask who on staff teaches cosmetic surgery, and make your first appointment with him or her. If there isn't such an institution nearby, ask your personal physician for a recommendation. If your physician has no recommendations, you can call the American Academy of Facial Plastic and Reconstructive Surgery at (800) 332–3223 and ask them for a list of members practicing in your area. All of these are great ways to shop for a cosmetic surgeon.

How to Interview a Cosmetic Surgeon

Notice I used the word *interview*. Your first appointment with a cosmetic surgeon is an interview—a fact-finding session. What you want to find out is not only how much the surgeon knows, but how he or she interacts with you, how compassionate the surgeon is, how much time he is willing to spend with you, how much information he is willing to give you, and also how much the surgeon charges for the procedure you are interested in. The first interview does not have to be the last. You can leave and think about what you've learned. You can discuss with your personal physician what transpired during your first interview. After you've done that, you can schedule another interview session and ask an entirely new set of questions. Once you have asked all the pertinent questions, you still need to talk to at least one other cosmetic surgeon for confirmation or for another opinion, even if you are comfortable with this surgeon.

The interview process is not an easy one, and it can be expensive, but it is essential. This is not the place to bargain hunt or cut costs. You would be surprised how many surgeons spend a significant amount of time in the interview process. They may talk to a woman several times over a year or two before the actual surgery takes place. When this time and care are taken, the likelihood is increased that you will make a better decision, have a better relationship with the surgeon you eventually select, and be more satisfied with the results of the surgery.

If I could, I would insist that you ask the following questions the first time you meet with a cosmetic surgeon.

1 Are you certified by the American Board of Plastic Surgery? (This is basic information to confirm that the doctor is indeed specially trained in cosmetic surgery; your answer may be framed and hanging on the wall.)

2 Are you a member of the American College of Surgeons? (This board is a prestigious association and indicates approval from the surgeon's peers; again, you can check the wall.)

3 Are you a staff member of an accredited hospital, teaching hospital, or university? (If the doctor teaches other doctors how to do cosmetic surgery, that is a very good sign.)

4 How long have you been in practice? (Although length of time may not be an indicator of quality, it is an indicator of experience.)

5 What types of cosmetic surgery do you perform most often? (If you are looking for an eye tuck, you may not want to go to a surgeon who does mostly breast implants or liposuction.)

6 Can you show me the results of previous surgeries, including before-and-after pictures? (What you want to pay attention to is the overall appearance and the placement of scars. Seeing results is a powerful determining factor.)

7 May I talk to any of your patients to get their feedback about their surgery experience? (Hearing the experiences of other patients is greatly reassuring.)

8 What steps do you take to keep the face from looking masklike or surprised? (Be sure you know what you *don't* want from your cosmetic surgery, and make sure your surgeon is concerned about the same things.)

9 What procedures do you use to eliminate as much of the sagging and wrinkling from around my eyes and jaw area as possible? (You want your surgeon to be realistic in this area, but you also don't want to be left with more aged skin then necessary. Looking at the before-and-after pictures of other patients will also help you in this regard.)

10 Do you think I am a good candidate for the procedure I am interested in? (You want an honest evaluation and a summary of what you can expect.)

11 What are the possible complications of the type of surgery I'm interested in? (The list for this question had better be long, or your doctor is giving you the bum's rush and a distorted picture of reality. Complications are indeed rare, but they do happen, and I've talked to enough women who have had problems to know that they can range from minor to severe. Knowing all your risks will only make you a better, more self-assured patient. If the surgeon doesn't want you to be well informed, find yourself another surgeon.)

12 What will I need to do after the surgery? How long will my recovery be and what can I expect in terms of bruising or bandages? Will I need someone to look after me for a period of time? How long will I have to miss work?

Although the process I am suggesting is a long one, I know that it culminates in finding a surgeon you can feel justifiably secure with. It sure is a much better evaluation process than calling up a friend and asking, "So do you know who did Elaine's face-lift? It looks great?"

Collagen Injections

Compared to a face-lift, collagen injections are a relatively nonintrusive way to rid the face of wrinkles. It can be done in a short period of time in your dermatologist's or plastic surgeon's office for a relatively small expense and potentially little risk. This technique can net an amazing long-term, although temporary, change in the appearance of wrinkles on the face.

One of the major reasons a wrinkle or scar occurs is because the collagen and elastin—the support fibers of the skin—break down. Collagen injections—not collagen creams—can temporarily rebuild the skin's depleted collagen supply by reintroducing pure collagen into the skin. When collagen is injected into your skin a high percentage of it merges with your own collagen, taking on the characteristics of the surrounding tissue. Injectable collagen actually becomes a functioning part of your skin.

Collagen injections can greatly diminish laugh lines, frown lines, some acne scars, and vertical lines from around the mouth. This nonsurgical, injectable method of raising the crevices formed by sun damage or scarring is truly remarkable, with relatively rare negative side effects. Collagen injections do not, however, replace what a face-lift or eye tuck can do. For example, collagen injections cannot be used on sagging jowls or drooping eyelids. They are also never used for the treatment of the lines under the eyes, "ice pick"-type acne scars, or scars with sharply defined edges. But for the lines and scars it can be used on, the results will blow you out of the water.

What age group can consider having collagen injections? If you have a wrinkle or scar that is suitable for injection, how old you are makes no difference. The entire procedure takes place in your doctor's office with relatively little discomfort and in a remarkably short period of time. The results are immediate. The cost can vary widely from doctor to doctor, regardless of the type of collagen used. Also, the skill of the doctor can vary greatly, depending on his or her experience specifically with collagen injections. You may have to shop around before you find a dermatologist or cosmetic surgeon who is well versed in the procedure. There is a toll-free number you can call to one of the companies that produces injectable collagen. The company is called the Collagen Corporation and the number is (800) 227–4004. They can give you information on physicians in your area who are most familiar with injectable collagen.

Once you make your decision to have collagen injections, the next step is for your doctor to make reasonably certain you are not allergic to the substance that will be used. Some people react negatively to injected collagen. The reaction will most likely not be serious or permanent. A small rash or swelling is the most typical reaction in those who are indeed sensitive to injected collagen. It is essential that your physician perform a skin-sensitivity test by injecting the collagen into a patch of skin on your arm. The doctor needs to check the test site in three days and then again in one month to be relatively sure there is no reaction. However, the patch test is not 100 percent accurate. A small percentage of people who have no reaction to the patch test still have an allergic reaction to the collagen.

There are other complications that can arise from collagen injection, and although they are considered rare, you should still be familiar with all the risks. It is possible for the doctor to place the needle in the skin incorrectly, causing damage to a blood vessel; the injected collagen may show through on the surface of the skin as a raised white bump that can persist for a few weeks or months; the injection site can become hard, red, or develop a rash that can last for a few weeks or months; and those people who have had herpes simplex where the injection is given may experience a herpes flare-up. All of these issues and more must be discussed with your doctor before you begin treatment.

When the patch test is done and there have been minor or no side effects, you can make your appointment to begin treatment. The results are immediate. Presto! After you leave your doctor's office, for a period of six months to one year, depending on your skin and the type of collagen that is used, no more wrinkles will appear—until the next injection. The need for repeated treatment is due to the nature of the injected collagen. The injected collagen behaves so much like your own collagen it is eventually depleted and needs to be rebuilt to maintain the desired effect.

The Crusty Matter of Face Peels

I should tell you from the start that I am not in favor of most facial peels. I feel that much of the information available about them is at best misleading. Anything you've read or any physician who tells you there aren't some fairly serious side effects of peeling the top layers of skin away, and in some cases the living layers of skin as well, would be avoiding the truth. The claim is that chemical face peels can either temporarily or permanently (depending on the type of chemical used) get rid of wrinkles and some skin discolorations. Quite a claim for applying what some have called fluid face fire to the skin!

There are several different types of chemical peels available. The categories of peels are *light*, *medium*, and *deep*. Alphahydroxy acids are chemical peels in the *light*-peel category. A dermatologist applies the acid solution directly to your face with a cotton swab or spatula. This relatively lightweight acid stays on the skin for several minutes. The solution is then neutralized with a mixture of baking soda and water. After this is removed your skin will be visibly red and burning. The irritation will continue for approximately one week. During this time your skin will peel off in thick layers. The claim is that once the shedding stops the skin will look smoother for up to three to six months. There is nothing about this peel that eliminates wrinkles. The severe irritation causes a semipermanent swelling of the skin that can make skin look smoother. The length of time is also not one you can count on. The results last only as long as the skin remains irritated. Once the skin returns to normal, it is suggested you do it again and again and again. This becomes a fairly costly procedure over time, totaling an average of $1,000 for three to four treatments over the course of a year—as well as about three to four weeks of rest over a year's time, because you can't go anywhere while your face is peeling away, which isn't the most attractive look in the world.

The next type of chemical face peel available is called trichloroacetic acid, and it is considered to be a *light* to *medium* peel. This acid is more toxic than the alphahydroxy acids, but the basic procedure at your doctor's office is about the same. The acid is applied to the skin with a cotton swab or spatula and is left on the face for approximately fifteen to sixty minutes depending on the degree of peel you are trying to achieve. The deeper peel requires local anesthesia. After the acid is neutralized the skin will burn intensely and look fiery red. The face is left totally raw and peeled. Within a day or two the skin will begin to develop crusty scabs. Over the next week or two the skin will go through a startling and uncomfortable peeling process. After about a month the redness will subside. The claim is that the skin will look smooth and wrinkle free for a period of four to ten months. But the skin hasn't lost a wrinkle; it is simply so swollen that the wrinkles are temporarily plumped out. It is suggested you repeat this process once every six months to a year. The cost for the trichloroacetic acid peel is about $300 to $4,000, depending on the extent of the peel and what the doctor feels the consumer will pay. Add to that the time you would have to be out of commission and this becomes a lot of pain, as well as money and time, only to have your wrinkles return in a few months.

Another chemical used to provide a *medium* peel is resorcinol. A ten percent solution is applied to the face in much the same manner as for the ones mentioned above. The turmoil the skin goes through is also the same as above: red, burned skin that scabs and peels over a period of one to two weeks. After the redness and peeling subside the skin initially looks smoother, but the wrinkles return after a period of time and then it is suggested you go through the process again. The price is about $500 and the recovery time is about two to three weeks.

Phenol, used for *deep* peeling, is the strongest form of chemical peel available. Unfortunately, deep peeling is often referred to as a *nonsurgical face-lift*. Do not be misled. Although no skin is cut, the pain and recovery time are considerable. This is a very intrusive, potentially dangerous procedure. Calling a deep peel *nonsurgical* makes it sound like a piece of cake, and nothing could be further from the truth. Phenol is applied in the doctor's office under local or general anesthesia. Once the phenol solution is applied, the skin is masked with tape to increase the burning power of the chemical. The procedure can last up to four hours, during which time the skin is literally liquefied. Some patients go home still masked and are told to sleep upright and minimize any and all facial movements. Eating is done only through a straw to enable the face to remain as still as possible. In a day or two the patient returns to the doctor's office, where the tape is removed. The skin underneath resembles a severe burn—oozing, severely swollen, and red. The patient is given instructions as to how to reduce the chances of infection at home. Over the next week the skin forms a hard crust, which slowly peels away. In a week or two the patient is able to leave the house. The intense redness can persist for up to six months. The claim is that the lines and scars can be eliminated for years. The cost is about $2,500 to $5,000, and the recovery time can be as long as two months.

There are several risks associated with medium and deep peels that you should know about. They include infection that can cause severe scarring, persistent redness, sun sensitivity, irregular pigmentation or discoloration, and potential disfigurement. Phenol peels can also cause kidney failure and heart irregularities. All chemical peels are dependent on the skill of the doctor performing the procedure. But even when the doctor is highly qualified, it is almost impossible to control the depth of the peel. Skin thickness varies from person to person and can vary from one part of the face to another. Accounting for those variations in skin thickness is precarious, and the result can be a peel that penetrates too deeply in one section of the face, damaging that area instead of improving it.

Given the risks associated with the use of phenol, resorcinol, and the stronger dose of trichloroacetic acid, there are many overwhelming reasons, in my opinion, to avoid these procedures. The light peels have less risk associated with them, but there are still risks and the benefits are at best temporary.

Is there ever a reason to do a chemical peel of any kind? The only definite change you can probably count on from a medium to deep peel is a reduction in superficial acne scars, fine lines, and brown sun spots. Is it worth the risk? That is a question you need to discuss with your physician. However, there is a lot of money to be made from these procedures, and the physicians doing them are not necessarily an objective source of information. If you are still interested in looking further into this, be sure to talk with your personal physician, or find a doctor who is familiar with chemical peels but does not personally perform them.

Chapter Five
Settling the Score With Your Acne

Acne is a Four-Letter Word

The cosmetics industry spends a good portion of its $16 billion revenues getting you to associate skin care with wrinkle-free creams, emolients, and moisturizers. It spends another large segment of its ad budget touting acne products. It is this expenditure that I am personally most concerned about because I can attest to the fact that cosmetic acne "medications" don't work. At least when you buy almost any moisturizer you can be reasonably sure that it will take care of your dry skin. The same cannot be said for acne products. I grew up with acne and I am still struggling with it today. I spent years using every available product you can imagine to "dry up" blemishes and get rid of my acne. None of the products ever worked, and judging from the thousands of letters I've received over the years, a large number of consumers feel the same way. Even dermatologists will agree that over-the-counter acne products work for only about 40 percent of the people who try them. Running around the acne merry-go-round of products is an irritating, tiresome game, and you usually still end up breaking out.

Growing up with acne wasn't easy. Before I went to bed at night the one thing I remember praying for was to have good skin. There were times my skin was worse than others, but it was always on the edge of disaster. My humiliation knew no bounds. Big ones right in the center of my forehead or on the tip of my nose giving way to a collection of medium to small ones driving me nuts on my cheek or chin. My memory has registered that I was the only one I knew with acne. I know that can't be true, but the feeling was one of distinct isolation. And it was lonely. Who cared that my acne, as far as I was concerned, was a terminal disease? From the age of eleven, along with the advent of puberty, my hormones and whatever other factors were in play ruled my face and much of my self-confidence.

Back then I thought that acne was my fault. My face just wasn't clean enough, so I washed it often, sometimes too hard, in the vain hope that my face would clear up. None of that was due to youthful ignorance: it was the message all of us received from ads, salespeople, and the products themselves. At one time I was prescribed to use a bar soap, an astringent, Cleocin lotion (an antibiotic lotion), Retin-A, and a Buff Puff. Within a matter of days my face felt like it was on fire. I went to bed in tears. But I still thought the more it burned the more all these things must be working to clear up my acne. The burning was a sign to me that it must be killing whatever it was that was making me break out. If only someone had told me that acne and blackheads had nothing to do with having dirty skin, and that clearing it up had nothing in the world to do with pain, I would have been grateful. Well, at least now I know better.

For most of us who suffer with acne, past and present, it is an embarrassment that all the makeup in the world can't keep secret. The worst thing is that most blemishes don't occur on the sides of the face near the hairline—noooo!—they occur in the center of the face, right in the line of vision. If you're like me, you don't want to understand acne, you want to get rid of it. Even doctors don't entirely know why acne happens—why one person gets acne but another doesn't, or why a dozen pores on your face break out at the same time but not all of them. They know that hormones play a large part—teenagers break out more than adults, women break out more before they get their periods—but they aren't exactly sure why. Why the face erupts in such unsightly, swollen, red or white bumps or dozens of small black or white circular dots is still, to some degree, a mystery.

What I will try to do over the next few paragraphs is give you an overview of the different forms of blemishes, some reasons why they may occur, and, hopefully, what you can do about them. Bear with me—some of this isn't a pretty picture.

Understanding Acne and Blackheads

There are three components to the formation of blemishes: oil production, skin cell turnover, and bacteria. I've already discussed oil production page 64 and cell turnover page 56, but let me tell you how they can affect acne.

The oil in the oil gland (pore) is not a liquid, it is a semi-hard, whitish, waxlike substance underneath the surface of the skin that liquifies as it comes to the surface. In normal skin the oil flow is minimal and spreads, in an almost imperceptible layer, evenly over the surface of the face. For those who have oily skin that breaks out, the oil is greatly overproduced and cannot flow freely from the pore. The reason the oil flow gets blocked has to do with cell turnover.

Cell turnover is the process of skin cells moving from the lower layers of skin, where they are generated, to the skin's surface, where they die and are eventually shed. The oil gland itself, even though it is imperceptible to the eye, is also lined with skin cells that go through this same process. For those with normal skin, the skin cells that are being produced within the oil gland are shed along with the oil. The skin cells on the surface of the face are shed easily when the face is washed.

For those with oily skin, the skin cells on the surface are kept from shedding adequately by the heavy, sticky flow of oil. These blocked surface skin cells can also fill the pore and cause it to become clogged. There are also skin cells that are being shed by the lining of the oil gland, that cannot flow out of the pore along with the oil because the buildup of oil and dead surface skin cells holds them back, causing further blockage. If enough oil and blocking skin cells are mixed together, a plug is created, and when the opening of the pore is extremely tiny, a whitehead develops. As the oil and dead skin cells continue to build up there are several things that can happen to the whitehead: it can continue on to become a blackhead or a pimple. (A whitehead and a pimple are two different things.)

A blackhead is formed when the opening of the pore becomes stretched by the continued backup of the oil (remember, the oil in the pore is semi-hard) from the blockage caused by the dead skin cells from the surface of the skin and from within the oil gland. The color inside the stretched, clogged pore becomes black because of the buildup of the brown pigment cells called melanin that color the skin and also because of the chemical reaction that occurs when the exposed oil oxidizes with the air. A whitehead, a clogged pore that is not stretched open and thus has not been exposed to the air, appears white under the skin instead of dark.

The third component of a blemish forming is bacteria. All pores have bacteria living inside them. That is normal. The bacteria multiply beyond the normal range only when there is no oxygen around for them to breathe. A blocked, closed pore prevents air from getting into the pore, which encourages the breeding of this particular type of bacteria. When these bacteria start growing inside a pore that is backed up with oil and dead skin cells, you have the perfect environment for a pimple.

A pimple is produced when the blockage of oil and dead skin cells inside the oil gland gets to the point where the pressure literally explodes the oil gland. The ruptured oil gland allows the oil to spread into the surrounding skin structure, swelling the tissue. But because the oil inside the pore is hard, the swelling creates a hard, red bump on the face. What turns this swollen, red bump into a pimple is the presence of bacteria inside the pore.

The bacteria that have been nicely multiplying inside the clogged, closed pore (whitehead) start feeding on the oil. The bacteria continue to grow (multiply) because they don't have air and they have lots of oil to eat. This proliferation of bacteria inside the clogged pore creates the final stages of a pimple. The increasing bacteria are seen by the body as a problem, and the result is a rush of white blood cells to the lesion to fight the invaders. Now you have a full-fledged pimple filled with hard oil and white pus surrounded by swollen, inflamed skin.

The different sizes of acne lesions have various names; *papules* are the smallest lesions, *pustules* are the next largest, and *nodules* or *cysts* are the most severe and painful of the group. How severe a case of acne you develop also has names: *acne vulgaris*, *acne conglobata*, and *acne fulminans*. If you have severe, chronic acne comprised of nodules and cysts, you will want to see your dermatologist for treatment. I have little advice for severe acne sufferers that will really make a difference. But for those of you who break out with papules or pustules, there are things you can do to alleviate the condition, either in conjunction with your dermatologist's recommendations or on your own. If you are under the care of a dermatologist, you will always want to check with him or her before you do anything new or different to your skin.

Acne Myths

Myth 1. "Only teenagers get acne." I thought that until I turned thirty and it was still there. After the age of thirty I became used to the idea that my tendency to break out wasn't ever going to go away. I was going to grow old and wrinkle, and under my wrinkles there would be pimples. For those of us who break out, it's just part of life, something to accept to a certain extent and to fight, but differently than we did in the past.

Women and men between eleven and fifty can suffer from acne. It tends to be a problem equally distributed between both sexes during adolescence, with teenage boys having a slightly higher incidence of acne. As we get older the likelihood of men being plagued with post-puberty acne is less than it is for women. That's probably because of the volatility of female hormones, but there is little medical understanding of why hormones play a role in acne. It is known, however, that they do. If the medical powers that be had asked me, I could have told them that, too. Like clockwork, since I was eleven, I break out one week before I get my period.

Myth 2. "Don't squeeze." This is not a fun topic, but someone's got to handle it. Whether or not you use all of the skin care suggestions I recommend for acne and whether or not you use the products available at the drugstore or the department store, once you get a pimple and you don't remove what's inside, it will take twice as long to heal no matter what else you do. The skin is swollen, red, and painful because of what is inside the pore. Depending on the severity of the lesion, when you remove the oil (wax) and white blood cells (pus) that have built up inside the pimple, the swelling will go away almost immediately. The more severe the blemish, the more difficult it will be to remove. Whoever told you that squeezing blemishes would automatically cause scarring was 100 percent wrong, although it is true that improperly squeezing a blemish can cause damage. The method you use to squeeze the blemish is important.

I'm not the first person who has suggested that you have to open a lesion and remove what is inside to get rid of it, but I might be one of the first to describe exactly how you should go about it. Those of you who aren't interested in a graphic description of how to do this can skip to the next section. For those of you who are interested, the-blow-by-blow follows.

1 Squeeze blemishes only after washing the face and preferably after massaging with baking soda and using the three percent hydrogen peroxide. The baking soda will help remove any skin that might be covering the pore's opening.

2 Be sure the face is completely dry.

3 You can use your fingers covered with tissues or not; whichever is easiest for you is fine.

4 Be sure that your fingers are placed evenly on either side of the lesion around the borders of the reddest area.

5 Begin squeezing with even pressure ever so gently in a downward direction and then slowly move in toward the center of the lesion with a final gentle push up. The operative words here are *even pressure* and *gentle*.

6 If the blemish does not give easily, stop squeezing and try again. You may want to try placing your fingers at a different angle around the blemish before you try squeezing again. Never try squeezing more than twice. Oversqueezing can damage the surrounding skin tissue, and that is what causes scabs and scarring.

7 Never try to pick or scratch the blemish open. This will also cause scabs and scarring, and healing will take even longer than if you had left it alone.

How to Fight Acne Peaceably

In Chapter Two I discussed the skin care routine I recommend for someone with oily skin and acne. Now let me explain why I think it can work for acne. I recommend washing with the Cetaphil Lotion or a foaming face wash to keep the irritation on the skin to an absolute minimum. The reason for this is that too much irritation further inflames and swells the skin, which only serves to make the acne worse. What color is acne? Red. What color does overirritated skin become? Redder. Treating the skin gently can help prevent the acne from getting worse. The argument for using a strong, irritating cleanser on acned skin is to help get all the oil off and help exfoliate the skin. I agree that exfoliating the skin is essential in the treatment of acne, and getting the oil off the face is equally important, but there is a level of how much the skin can take. A cleanser should indeed remove all the oil, but as gently as possible. The next step, and only the next step, is where you help the skin to shed some of these backed up skin cells. You can't rip acne off the face, so overcleansing doesn't help anything.

The reason baking soda is effective in fighting acne is because it helps exfoliate the dead skin cells from the surface of the face. The fewer dead skin cells sticking together and building up, the less chance they have of blocking the pore's opening. Baking soda is all you need to help exfoliate the skin. Depending on your skin type, you should use the baking soda once or twice a day either directly on the skin or mixed with the Cetaphil Lotion.

The three percent hydrogen peroxide solution is used on the face for several reasons. First, because three percent hydrogen peroxide solution is an effective disinfectant, it can help to kill the bacteria inside the pore that is causing the pimple to form. Because the three percent hydrogen peroxide solution is not irritating to the skin surface it does this without further damaging the skin or stimulating more oil production. Second, three percent hydrogen peroxide solution can help reverse the oxidation of the clogged pore and make the dark color lighter. The last reason is that three percent hydrogen peroxide solution can help calm down the swelling of the skin.

The milk of magnesia used as a facial mask absorbs the excess oil that is in the pore. Milk of magnesia absorbs a great deal of oil and it doesn't irritate the skin.

This basic rationale for dealing with acne is not new. Many skin care routines and products on the market are based on the same theory as the one I've described above: clean the face, exfoliate the skin, kill the bacteria inside the pore, and do whatever you can to reduce the oil flow. The difference is that many over-the-counter remedies for acne, even though they may contain ingredients that kill bacteria, exfoliate the skin, and degrease the surface of the face, severely irritate the skin at the same time. If you can accomplish practically the same results with my routine as you can with over-the-counter acne medications, without irritating the skin, why not do it the gentle way? Acne is already red and irritated; it would be nice for a change to do something for the skin that doesn't make it more red and irritated, something that doesn't create an additional skin problem at the same time—dry skin.

Note: *Please be aware that nothing gets rid of blackheads and acne 100 percent. What I'm suggesting is a way to control acne to a degree and calm down the skin at the same time. Reducing oil production is the primary method of curing acne, which can only be done medically with the prescription oral drug called Accutane, which I'll get to next.*

By the way, an occasional pimple now and then does not make a case of acne. I can't tell you how many women with one pimple on their chin have informed me they have an appointment with their dermatologist that week. That's truly overreacting. What happens to skin sometimes, regardless of skin type, is that it breaks out, and there isn't much a doctor, a cosmetics company, or the routine I've explained here can do to change that. Hopefully, what I've recommended is a course of action you can take when you do break out that will help retard the process.

If you choose to fight acne by making an appointment with a dermatologist, let me go over a few of the prescriptions that you may be given to take into battle with you. They are Retin-A, Cleocin lotion, Accutane, Retin-A, and oral antibiotics. One at a time I'll review what they are and what they can do.

The Radical Acne Cure—Accutane

Accutane is an oral drug that can perform miracles for many people with severe acne or chronic cystic acne. Accutane is a derivative of vitamin A (just like Retin-A) that is taken by mouth in pill form. If you have severe acne, please discuss its use with your physician. Oral doses of Accutane literally stop the body's production of oil. With no oil present there can't be any clogged pores. Treatment usually lasts anywhere from a few months to a year, with the average length of time being six months. The best part is that once you stop taking the Accutane, for some reason the acne does not return. Doctors are not exactly sure why that happens, but it does. The cure rate is astounding. Unfortunately, after heaping all this glory upon Accutane, I must also warn you that Accutane is associated with very serious and potentially dangerous side effects.

Because of the potential problems associated with Accutane, it is only recommended in extreme chronic cases of acne; it is not recommended for your basic, everyday, run-of-the-mill, acute cases of acne. Acute acne differs from chronic acne in the intensity, size, and frequency of blemishes. *Acute acne* describes small to medium-size blemishes that may cause minor scarring but don't disfigure the skin. *Chronic acne* refers to large, recurring blemishes that can permanently distort the shape and appearance of the skin.

Be sure to completely go over Accutane's side effects with your physician, step by step. You need to know what you can do for any of the complications that may occur before you make a decision to use it. Accutane can cause brittle bones, backaches, liver and kidney problems, very dry skin, and blood cell problems. It can also cause miscarriages and fetal deformities. This is a very serious drug that needs to be dealt with cautiously.

It would be a good idea for you to know how long you will need to be on Accutane and how much the entire therapy will cost. Accutane therapy can be very expensive. You will also need to make repeat visits to the doctor to check on your progress, monitor your blood count, and keep track of what is happening to you physically. Accutane is not something you would ever want to take without ongoing supervision from your dermatologist. You may want to find out ahead of time if your medical insurance covers Accutane therapy. For those of you who can use it, it can indeed cure cases of acne that, prior to the days of Accutane, used to leave many with no hope of avoiding disfigured, scarred facial skin.

Remember: *Accutane can cause serious problems for pregnant women. Miscarriages and severe birth defects have been associated with taking Accutane. If you are pregnant or are considering having a baby you should not be taking Accutane. Accutane carries a strong warning label with this information. When Accutane was first made available, many women and doctors ignored these warnings and the results were tragic. Doctors frequently prescribed Accutane to young people, who are not always careful or aware of the responsibilities of birth control. And, of course, a woman might start taking the drug before being aware that she is pregnant. That is a risk. If you are sincerely interested in trying Accutane to help eliminate the disfiguring effects of chronic acne, then it is essential you either consider using some type of birth control or abstain from sexual relations altogether until the Accutane therapy is complete.*

Retin-A For Acne

In Chapter Three I discussed at length using Retin-A on sun-damaged skin. It is, however, foremost a viable option for many women with acute acne. When I first tried Retin-A when I was 18 years old I personally found it too irritating to use, and I have received many letters from other women who have also tried Retin-A for acne and found it too irritating. After trying Retin-A again, for sun-damaged skin this time, and using a skin care routine that helped relieve much of the irritation, I found that even though I liked the way my skin felt while I was using it, I still had the same problems with acne. But that doesn't mean it won't work for you. It is definitely worth a try.

Chapter Three on Retin-A, which deals mainly with using Retin-A for sun-damaged skin, is valid information for someone with acne. Basically I recommend following the same precautions and the same gradual incremental increases for both sun-damaged skin and acne. The reason for this as I mentioned before is because Retin-A can cause mild to severe skin irritation regardless of skin type. Another reason why our experiences with Retin-A may have been uncomfortable is because of the strength of the prescription that was doled out. Doctors may automatically prescribe the strongest percentage gel or liquid form of the Retin-A for their patients who have oily skin. Many physicians disagree with my concern about alcohol or irritants on acned skin types. They may feel that alcohol increases the absorption of the Retin-A into the skin, which it does, thereby accelerating the affect on the skin. This may indeed be beneficial for some forms of acne. I would still suggest that you can build to this level slowly and avoid any additional irritants as you progress to the stronger dosage. If you suggest to your doctor that you start with the weaker cream base, increasing over a period of time to the liquid or gel, you may be surprised how open he or she may be to your suggestion. If your skin reacts favorably, you can always move to the stronger percentages next time you need a refill, and more frequent applications.

For some acned skin, to achieve the maximum benefit, depending on your doctor's recommendation, it is best to use the Retin-A (regardless of the strength) twice a day if you can tolerate it. To build up your tolerance follow the instructions on page 108.

Cleocin Lotion and Oral Antibiotics for Acne

The topical antibiotic Cleocin lotion is a very popular prescription that dermatologists use hand in hand with Retin-A. It consists of the antibiotic clindamycin dissolved in alcohol which is then used as an astringent. Technically the Cleocin lotion works along the same theoretical line as the three percent hydrogen peroxide or the five percent or ten percent benzyl peroxide. All three get into the pore (sebaceous gland) and work to kill the bacteria that are hanging out in there helping to create your blemishes. Supposedly the Cleocin lotion, because it contains a strong antibiotic and is suspended in alcohol, is considered to do a more thorough job than the three percent peroxide or the five percent and ten percent benzyl peroxides. For some acned skin types, that is indeed true. As you already know, I think there are too many problems with using alcohol on the skin for such use to be justified. While obtaining an effective disinfectant, you also acquire an incredibly strong—and I mean strong—irritant. Whatever the benefit of the antibiotic, you may also develop skin that becomes inflamed and dried out.

An adjustment to the Cleocin prescription can solve this problem. Cleocin lotion can be made primarily with Cetaphil Lotion. What the dermatologist can do is write a special prescription that instructs the pharmacist to dissolve the clindamycin tablets in a minimal amount of alcohol and then mix that solution with the Cetaphil. The lotion is mostly the very gentle, nonirritating Cetaphil and the antibiotic itself, with little to no residual alcohol. Now that you know more clearly what your options are you can make the gentle choices on your own or you can encourage your doctor to treat your skin more gently from the start.

Another standard prescription for most acne patients is oral antibiotics. For the most part, many people taking oral antibiotics experience an immediate, positive difference in their skin. You may still break out, but the frequency and amount that take place will be reduced. The negative thing about taking oral antibiotics is that it isn't great to stay on a prescription medication for extended periods of time. The possible side effects of taking oral antibiotics are stomach problems, yeast infections, teeth becoming discolored and adapting to the antibiotic so it is no longer effective. For the most part, the side effects stop once you discontinue usage, except for adapting to the antibiotic. In that case the physician simply prescribes a different one and the positive, and possibly the negative, results can begin all over again. Because of the positive results of taking oral antibiotics, many people are willing to suffer with the side effects, and most dermatologists will tell you that these aren't that bad. I'm not sure I agree, but I would be hard put to deny the benefits. While I was taking antibiotics, chronic yeast infections were a monthly struggle and were simply not worth it. You will have to weigh the pros and cons for yourself before you choose what to do. There is no easy answer with this one.

What to Ask Your Doctor

If you find that the skin care routine I'm suggesting for acne doesn't work and you decide to see a dermatologist, keep the notion of gentle firmly implanted in your mind and evaluate your skin care options with the doctor from this point of view. Here is a list of questions and ideas that can help when you go in for your appointment and the doctor recommends some of the things we've been talking about.

1 If at the time of the appointment you have serious questions about the prescriptions or products you've been given, talk to the doctor or nurse. The nurse often has very good information and is sometimes more patient than the doctor.

2 Ask the doctor what you're supposed to do when irritation occurs. Hopefully, the doctor will give you a weaker prescription or tell you to cut back the frequency of use.

3 Ask if you can skip a return office visit should you find you're not experiencing any difficulties. The doctor may let you check in by phone, and, if you're doing okay, call in to your druggist a prescription refill or a stronger percentage if needed at that time.

4 Be sure to get a thorough explanation of how the prescriptions you will be using can affect your skin in the sun. Read the instructions back to the doctor so that you are sure you understand everything.

5 Take notes while you are with the doctor and bring your questions with you. You don't want to leave the appointment feeling like you wished you had asked a dozen things you forgot to while you were there.

Summary:

Whether it is decided that you go on Accutane therapy or topical Retin-A and Cleocin lotion, it would be wise to use Cetaphil as your water-soluble cleanser when you wash your face. The major drawback to both these skin care prescriptions is that they can render the skin exceedingly dry and irritated. Cetaphil will clean the skin and not dry it out any further. You will find that most soaps on the market will leave your face painfully dry. The same is doubly true if you are using any products that contain alcohol. The combination of these prescriptions with soap (even so-called *nonirritating* soaps), scrubs, and alcohol-based cosmetics can ruin your face. I would encourage you to avoid anything on the face that can cause unnecessary irritation such as astringents, all bar soaps, washcloths, tissues, scrub products (at least not all over the face), facial masks, hot water, and any products that are designed to dry up acne.

A Just-In-Case Checklist

This is a practical checklist to make sure you've double-checked all the possible things that may be aggravating your acne besides your skin care routine. Although most acne is not solely caused by allergies to food or cosmetics, it can be made worse by both. (If I just look at a moisturizer—any moisturizer—I break out immediately.) To help avoid or at least somewhat curb those factors that could be compounding the problem, be aware that any of the following can be trouble for those of you who have severe to mild forms of acne.

1 *Allergies to milk fat or dairy products in general.* Although, generally speaking, diet *does not* affect acne, there are a few foods that have been known to cause skin reactions. Chocolate, however, is not one of them, unless of course it is milk chocolate and you have a problem with milk.

2 *Allergies to shellfish or nuts, or any other suspect foods or food groups.* If you are curious to see if a particular food group is the culprit, simply stop eating all forms of whatever it is you want to check out for two to three months and see what happens. If you stop for shorter periods of time and your skin clears up, that may be coincidence rather than fact. Your skin needs time to see what happens to it over the long haul. Doctors can perform allergy tests, too.

3 *Problems with fluoride in toothpastes, especially if you're just breaking out around your mouth and chin.* If you suspect this is true for you, check with your dentist and try brushing with baking soda and three percent hydrogen peroxide instead of toothpaste for a while and see what happens. The American Dental Association recommends the combination of baking soda and three percent hydrogen peroxide as a way to fight bacteria buildup in the mouth.

4 *Irritation from your partner's beard, particularly if you're just breaking out around the chin and mouth.* This is definitely a problem for women with sensitive skin.

5 *Not getting all your makeup off at night.* If you have a problem with blemishes and you sleep in your makeup, I assure you, you will have a bigger blemish problem in the morning.

6 *Certain cosmetics, such as foundations, moisturizers, or cream blushes*—especially if the lesions are occurring only where you use them. Test your sensitivity to any of these potential allergens by eliminating them one at a time and watching the results for a few months. It may make a marked difference in the appearance of your skin.

7 *Some shampoos, particularly those with conditioners.* Try a few different types of shampoos to see if your face is having more problems with one than the others.

Chapter Six
Creating a Makeup Wardrobe

A Makeup Wardrobe Just For You

Two major problems women have with makeup are choosing the right colors for their skin and discerning the differences between products. These problems need to be addressed, but they are only part of the picture. Before you choose specific makeup colors or products, it is important to have a clear picture of the makeup look and style you want to create. You wouldn't go shopping for a piece of clothing unless you knew what color and style of outfit you were going to wear with it. A cotton T-shirt would not complement a wool gabardine business suit. Nor would you get dressed before you had an idea of where you were going. You wouldn't put on a jogging suit to go to a formal dinner.

Color, style, and use are all essential elements of getting dressed, but they are also essential to putting together a great makeup look. Too often women shop or apply makeup with only one of these things in mind. Shopping for a lipstick or eyeshadow color independent of any other item in your makeup wardrobe is a mistake. Wondering where to put your blush or how to blend your foundation before you know why you should be wearing these things in the first place is also a common error. The primary way to improve your makeup shopping and makeup applying habits is to decide what kind of makeup wardrobe you want to create and then go about choosing compatible colors, products, and application techniques.

The things that affect the way you choose and wear makeup are the way you see yourself, how you want to be seen, what you do for a living, what you do in your leisure time, what colors are in your wardrobe, what style of clothing you are comfortable in, and how much time you are willing to spend creating a particular look. Those elements combine to set the course for choosing the right colors and products. Before we discuss whether you should be wearing brown eyeshadow or green eyeshadow or using liquid foundation or cream-to-powder foundation, it is essential to evaluate these other aspects of your makeup look.

Dress Your Face According to Your Image

The first part of this makeup self-analysis is to take a close look at yourself. How do you want to be seen? What do you do for a living? What occupies most of your time during the day? The external image you want to project in your business and personal life is what wearing makeup is all about. Too often we dress our faces without thinking about how it affects our image. The best example of this can be seen in the movie *Working Girl* with Melanie Griffith and Harrison Ford. If you've seen this movie, you probably noticed the dramatic change in Melanie's appearance as her character decides to become more "professional" in order to enhance her career aspirations. Besides the change in her wardrobe, I noticed the change in the way she wore her makeup. She decided that in order to look more "polished and together" she needed to soften her makeup look. The striking difference in her looks was a beautiful example of how makeup can affect the image you project.

Begin the process of choosing the image you want to project (and the one that works best for you) by examining the various possibilities. The following list includes nine basic images. Review the list and see which one describes you the best. Perhaps some of these can give you an idea how to approach the way you do your makeup (or get dressed) every morning in a more goal-oriented framework. Rather than just randomly selecting a lipstick, you may want to stop and consider not only whether it's the right color for the outfit you're wearing, but whether it is too soft, too sheer, too noticeable, too sexy, not sexy enough, or has enough flare to support the image you want to project. The problems that accompany how we apply our makeup can be solved once we come to understand ourselves better.

Images

Image 1. The Artist

Profile: The Artist is one who is daring, creative, and dramatic, and wants to be recognized as such. New ideas that run the gamut from art to literature are the fire that keeps the Artist alive. Key words are *provocative, intriguing, imaginative,* and *talented.*

Artist career choices: Graphic artist, writer, novelist, entertainer, publicity manager, columnist, actress, dancer, dance instructor, choreographer, drama coach, art teacher, architect.

Makeup for the Artist: Makeup for the Artist needs to have the same flare as her personality. The eye design can be a bit more dramatic than the average or the lip color a bit more extravagant. Too little makeup or poorly applied makeup can make the Artist look more like a hippie than a fashion statement. On the other hand, there is also the risk that The Artist can get carried away and apply too much makeup and look overdone. Balance is the key word for the Artist when assembling a creative makeup wardrobe.

When it comes to clothing the Artist can appear more intriguing by adding an exotic scarf or handcrafted earrings to accessorize a traditional business suit. Only one or two clothing items are necessary to make a daring statement without overdoing it. The same is true for makeup. A subtle foundation, with soft blush and eyeshadow colors accented by a vivid lipstick or a dramatic eyeliner, can make the same dynamic impression without making the makeup more noticeable than the person.

Image 2. The Professional

Profile: No matter what else the Professional is doing, her true focus is on either advancing her career or trying to create one. The Professional is happiest when she is being productive and effective. *Self-assured*, *classic*, *successful*, and *sophisticated* are the words that best describe this individual.

Professional career choices: Any position within the corporate world that allows room for advancement (including the ultimate potential promotion to president or chairman of the board) or any entrepreneurial venture that promises to expand and grow.

Makeup for the Professional: Choosing a makeup wardrobe for the Professional is challenging because too much can be just as inappropriate as too little. The Professional, in order to be taken seriously and look good, needs a full makeup effect that is a happy medium between attractive and powerful. This is *not* the time to look sexy, or masculine. That is no easy task. A soft but colorful lipstick color, well-blended foundation, muted and contoured eye design, and pale blush are essential for a professional look. Any part that is too vivid or exaggerated will look out of place. Clothing poses the same balance problem. Power dressing is the rule of thumb for this image, yet this is a look that can easily turn into a uniform and become extremely masculine. A man's suit and shirt is for men, not women, but if you do wear a man's-style suit, opt for a more feminine silk blouse, nylons with a simple stylish design, and interesting medium-sized earrings to give it more flare. Don't lose yourself in the corporate image.

Image 3. The Athlete

Profile: The Athlete emphasizes being strong, moving easily, feeling healthy, and taking care of others at the same time. The term *athlete* is meant here not so much as a physical attribute as an attitude about life and well-being. In everything the Athlete does, whether it is work or play, the desire is to always be seen as one who cares about being physically capable and healthy. Casual is a style the Athlete loves because of how it facilitates approaching life with energy and comfort.

Athlete career choices: Nutritionist, health administrator, aerobics instructor, gym teacher, park managment, recreational specialist, occupational therapist or specialist, athletic trainer.

Makeup for the Athlete: Makeup is not a favorite part of the Athlete's wardrobe. Yet because the Athlete doesn't care too much for cosmetics in general, the tendency is for her to concentrate on only one facet of her makeup. The Athlete may choose to wear only mascara and or just foundation and blush, which leaves the rest of the face looking too plain. The rule here is tasteful, balanced simplicity. Athletes can easily get away with the minimum amount of makeup, but the minimum needs to be equal. A little mascara, soft blush, and a subtle shade of lipstick create a great daytime, casual look. Do not throw on blue eyeshadow and call it eye design.

Image 4. The Trendsetter

Profile: Simply stated, the Trendsetter knows what's going on, and you can tell by looking at her that her information is up-to-date and accurate. This is a person who loves being on the edge of whatever is happening. Fashion magazines or trade publications are essential to keeping abreast of industry forecasts and changes. Being one step ahead of everyone else is paramount to the Trendsetter and her success is gauged by counting the number of people who follow her example.

Trendsetter career choices: Fashion consultant, specialty salesperson, public relations director, advertising account executive, attorney, stockbroker, clothes buyer, interior designer, marketing consultant.

Makeup for the Trendsetter: To make this statement clearly and concisely with both clothing and makeup, your makeup should either be a full classic look, so that you're never out of style, or the most recent fashion designs the models in *Vogue* are sporting this season. If the latter is your preference, you will need to spend a lot of time at the fashion boutiques or at the cosmetics counters so you always have the latest fashion look. The Trendsetter can prove to be one of the more expensive images to create and maintain.

You also need to be cautious about being so up-to-date that you look out of place. For example, if you are always looking for makeup colors that are the latest rage, if they don't catch on, you have wasted money or looked strange for a while (brown blush is a good example of a fashion statement that never really caught on). When it comes to your makeup wardrobe, I would always vote for a basic classic look with only one element that is new and different, just to be on the safe side.

Image 5. The Educator

Profile: The Educator epitomizes experience, mastery, and knowledge. The Educator is also an excellent communicator—without communication skills no teacher can teach. The classroom is not the only forum for this well-informed woman; business consultants and professional speakers often project this image.

Educator Career Choices: Teacher, professor, company trainer, product specialist, systems analyst, author of how-to books, accountant, sociologist, education developer, printer, acquisitions editor, engineer, editor, publisher, librarian.

Makeup for the Educator: The Educator is the epitome of conservative good taste. Because she is accomplished in her field and as a result needs to share what she's learned, it is important to make the conservative style stand out more than usual. The best way to make this statement is with a subtle (soft colors), full (foundation, blush, contour, eyeshadows, eyeliner, lipstick, and mascara) makeup application. A simplified makeup look can look too plain and too much makeup can look out of place. Balance is essential for the Educator.

Image 6. The Diplomat

Profile: The Diplomat is the peacemaker in the world, the one who handles disputes and is always looking for the perfect compromise. Negotiating is a skill that is second nature to the Diplomat. This individual is concerned with what everyone else thinks so that she can negotiate with acumen and insight. The secret the Diplomat knows is how to mix discretion with conviction. If you need to get people to see your point of view, you must be sensitive to the needs of others without forgetting your own.

Diplomat career choices: Politician, public relations director, personnel manager, secretary, doctor, nurse, counselor, lobbyist, office manager, caterer, diplomat.

Makeup for the Diplomat: Your makeup should reflect confidence, but the colors should be soft and subtle to avoid distraction. You don't want to offend anyone with what you're wearing or how you look. The makeup style that best portrays this image is a soft business look, but never too slick or fashionable. Classic is the direction all the way. For clothing that means two-piece suits with formal fabric and construction.

Image 7. The Home Manager

Profile: The Home Manager is a woman whose life revolves primarily around her home, consisting of her home management and social responsibilities and the social responsibilities of her husband and children. The Home Manager must juggle a schedule of organizational and private interests, whether it be for charity, government concerns, children's school, or her spouse's business needs. There is a flare and vibrancy to this lifestyle that is simultaneously leisurely, accomplished, and hectic. Because the Home Manager is often an unsung heroine, it is important to acknowledge the freedom that comes with this lifestyle choice as one of its benefits instead of its stigma.

Home Manager career choices: The career has already been chosen, and it is more a lifestyle than a job. The details of how to make this lifestyle productive and enjoyable for you is the major goal and challenge.

Makeup for the Home Manager: There is no right look for this career, and that is a problem as well as a blessing. The tendency is to go from one extreme to the other—either too little makeup or too much. I've encountered many women who were only going out for lunch or to the grocery store wearing a full, elaborate makeup application—more than I sometimes wear on television. Because there are no job description constraints or promotion considerations, you are left considering only your own image needs. My recommendation is to stick with the basics and wear a casual makeup during the day and a more sophisticated makeup at night.

Image 8. The Retired Adult

Profile: There is no one description that applies to the Retired Adult. This is as varied a group of people as you can imagine, with a wide assortment of interests, skills, and aspirations. What these women tend to share in common is a concern about their quality of life. *Casual* and *leisurely* are the key words for the Retired Adult, and this is reflected in a less stressful, easygoing lifestyle.

Retired Adult career choices: Retired Adults either work part time or are fully retired. Once again, there is a wide variety of abilities and skills represented by this group. The only limitations tend to be health, desire and, at times, discrimination.

Makeup for the Retired Adult: This is an image with no guidelines when it comes to makeup. Either a simple daytime makeup if the schedule is leisurely or a full, or soft makeup application when business is at hand is appropriate. The only caution for the Retired Adult is the tendency to ignore makeup problems that occur as the face changes. For example, lipstick bleeding, foundation slipping into lines on the face, powder clinging to the surface, eyelids that are more difficult to line, declining vision that makes a smooth, even makeup application more challenging require your attention (and a magnifying mirror). This is a time when too much makeup can really look overdone. It is essential to adapt your makeup look as necessary. I will explain how to go about making those changes later in this chapter.

Image 9. The Student

Profile: The Student is in the process of learning how to create the life she wants. There is a great deal of independence and latitude for those in the midst of creating their lives. In spite of this freedom, the Student's schedule is hectic and the decisions made today can greatly affect tomorrow.

Student Career Choices: Anything the Student puts full effort into she can probably do well.

Makeup for the Student: Although the tendency is for the Student to take a laid-back attitude about her appearance, this is the perfect time to cultivate and practice different images to see how they fit.

Working with Your Image

What do you do with the image you've chosen? Be the way you want to be now. Slowly but surely invest in yourself. I know some of you are saying you can't afford to do this. That stumbling block doesn't apply here because money isn't an issue in this goal. How much you own isn't what makes image happen. No matter how much you spend or own—one lipstick, one blush, or two eyeshadows—if it doesn't say what you want it to say about you, you've wasted your money. Now when you shop, do so with a purpose, keeping in mind what image you want to project. Before you buy another lipstick or eyeshadow, consider whether or not it goes with the image you've chosen for yourself.

Why Is Buying the Right Makeup So Difficult?

In all fairness to the cosmetics industry, the colors, textures, and varieties of products they produce are generally wonderful, easy to use, and last a reasonable length of time. They do not melt in the hot sun or freeze during the winter when left in a makeup bag inside a car while you go shopping. They do not grow strange molds or fungus, despite the fact that some cosmetics will spend most of their lives in a hot, damp bathroom. The most important fact about today's makeup is that there is little risk of permanent damage to the skin or eyes. So what do I have to complain about if all of that is true? Funny you should ask!

Someone asked me once, why, if I was so upset with the cosmetics industry, didn't I just stop wearing makeup? That would be like asking Ralph Nader, if he was so angry with the automobile industry, why didn't he just stop driving a car and walk? Being angry with parts of the automobile industry doesn't necessarily mean Mr. Nader doesn't like to drive to get where he's going. He may, in fact, love to drive. It's just that while he's behind the wheel he wants to be assured that he's getting his money's worth in quality and safety. Makeup for me is the same thing. I enjoy the remarkable effects that can be created with makeup, but that doesn't mean I want to buy overpriced makeup that smears, flakes off, and is accompanied by overinflated claims. I only want to deal realistically with the products I buy to put on my face—nothing more and nothing less. And that is exactly the kind of information you will receive in this chapter.

I love being creative with makeup, but I will neither deny nor overstate the wonders and problems of putting the stuff on as they do at the cosmetics counters and in many beauty books and fashion magazines. My intention is to list in a very straightforward, matter-of-fact way the pros and cons of each type of makeup product and what it takes to apply it with ease. I will also explain why some products aren't worth bothering with at all and why some products are better than others. Once you know the positives and negatives, you will find making decisions about what to wear and how to wear it easier and less costly.

With that in mind, this next section explains the makeup application techniques and theories I have developed over the years. Having applied more than a few lipsticks that bled all over the place, and mascaras that made lashes brittle and spiked-looking, and foundations that have gone on heavy, orange, and streaky, I have a few opinions as to what works and what doesn't work. As a makeup artist, TV commentator, and a woman who definitely enjoys wearing the stuff, my priority is to be sure my makeup looks attractive without wasting time to achieve that appearance, which is what I am about to describe in detail.

Before You Start

Because makeup goes on poorly over unclean skin, it goes without saying that the first step in applying beautiful makeup is to start with a clean face. More often than not, after washing your face with a water-soluble cleanser and following it with an irritant-free toner or three percent hydrogen peroxide, depending on your skin type, you can start applying your makeup. Generally speaking, except for those women with dry skin, I rarely recommend wearing a moisturizer under your foundation. However, if you want to protect your face from the sun during the day, regardless of your skin type, and you are not wearing a foundation that contains an SPF of 15 or greater, then it is best to wear a sunscreen of SPF 15 or greater under your foundation. Other than that, for those women with normal to oily skin, it is unnecessary to wear a moisturizer under your foundation.

There is no purpose to using a moisturizer other than to smooth and lubricate dry skin. A moisturizer does not and cannot protect the face from a foundation, nor is that necessary in spite of what you will hear from cosmetics salespeople. There is nothing "bad" inside a foundation that your face needs to be protected from. It's a good selling gimmick but not the truth. Moisturizers are made to be absorbed into the skin, and once they are, to all intents and purposes they're gone, and they can't prevent anything else you put on the face from going where it wants. Whatever layer of protection you think you're applying when you put on a moisturizer is wiped away as you apply your foundation.

I know this idea of wearing a moisturizer only when you have dry skin borders on the radical, but in the long run it makes the most sense. What you might not know is that most water-based foundations contain exactly the same ingredients as your moisturizer, so it isn't necessary to double up products. By wearing a moisturizer and a water-based foundation at the same time, your face can become too slippery and the rest of your makeup will tend to slide right off, never having a chance to make it past lunch. If you feel a moisturizer helps your foundation go on smoother, there could be a problem in your application technique or the type of foundation you're using, which will be discussed in the section on foundations.

A good way to judge whether or not your skin needs moisturizer during the day under your makeup (separate from a sunscreen) is to notice how long your skin feels dry after you wash your face. Some amount of drying is typical immediately after you wash your face. If this feeling lasts for longer than thirty minutes, it is probably best to wear a moisturizer under your foundation. If your skin tends to feel extremely dry after you wash your face, then it is essential to wear a good moisturizer under your foundation. If your skin tends to become drier as the day goes by, that too is a good reason to wear a moisturizer.

Never Do More Than You Have To!

My first theory of makeup application is to never do more than you have to. Wearing a moisturizer under a water-based foundation is just one of the many steps in applying makeup that can easily be eliminated without affecting your overall makeup look in any way.

One of the things that happens frequently at the cosmetics counter is that the salesperson tells you you need an absurd number of products in order to be properly and attractively made up. My job is to make things less complicated, because more complicated doesn't mean you will look any better. If anything, a more complicated makeup routine can mean more mistakes, causing you to look overdone and wasting your time.

Speaking of doing too much, so-called submoisturizers, eyelid foundations, blemish cover-ups, and color correctors—to name a few—are all completely unnecessary. They complicate an otherwise simple process of applying makeup by requiring additional blending and having too many colors and products interact on the skin at the same time. Your foundation (and moisturizer, if you have dry skin) can quite nicely accomplish all the functions those extra products are supposedly designed to handle without any of the fuss and expense.

Submoisturizers or premoisturizers are a new breed of moisturizer on the cosmetics scene. You find them mostly in the higher-priced cosmetics lines. Perhaps those women who can afford to spend the money are more easily convinced to waste it. These products are sold rather convincingly as being needed "to prepare and help the skin absorb the moisturizer." There is nothing in these submoisturizers other than standard moisturizing ingredients or irritant-free toners. They do not prepare the skin in any way and they do not help the moisturizer to be absorbed any better. These products are definitely a waste of time and money.

Eyelid foundations are sold to the consumer to help eyeshadows stay in place longer. The eye area is indeed a tricky place to get color to last, but there are ways to make it stay without special eyelid foundations. Besides, most eyelid foundations have a very similar formula to regular face foundations. These two so-called different products can be almost the same thing packaged in different containers. Placing your face foundation on your eyelid and putting loose powder over it will perform the same function the special eyelid foundation was supposed to accomplish. Also, if you are having problems with your eyeshadows, smearing or slipping into the crease will be greatly reduced if you do not place a moisturizer on your eyelid.

Blemish cover-ups are sold to the consumer solely because of something I call acne anxiety. The promise that is conveyed by the name cover-up is that this product really can hide a blemish, and nothing could be further from reality. Most cover-ups are a heavier texture than your foundation and over a blemish will appear thick and obvious. And if the blemish cover-up doesn't match your foundation exactly (which most don't), it will look like a different layer of color (usually orange) placed over the blemish, bringing more attention to the very problem you are trying to hide. If the cover-up turns out to be the same color as your foundation, you will still end up placing too much extra makeup over the lesion. Your foundation all by itself is more than sufficient to do the job of covering the redness without bringing more attention to the area. I totally understand the desire to want these facial sore spots to disappear. Unfortunately, there is only so much you can do to cover up a blemish before you start making matters worse.

Color correctors are those bottles of pink, lavender, or yellow liquids that are meant to be worn under your foundation to alter skin color. These little gems are hard to find anymore, but some cosmetics lines are steadfast in making you believe you need them. The notion is that if your skin is pink or ruddy in color you need to tone that down with a yellow-tinted color corrector. If your skin is olive or sallow in color you would use the pink or lavender color corrector to change that. Interesting concept, but totally a waste of time—these products can't do what they say they can do.

The ingredients listings for most color correctors are very similar to those for moisturizers, which means they are easily absorbed into the skin. Once they are absorbed, you are left with a slight tint of pink, lavender, or yellow on the face. Supposedly this means you have now changed your skin tone for the better. In fact, once the liquid has been absorbed, the result is so minor as to have no real effect on skin tone at all. For the sake of argument, though, let's say there is a noticeable effect. The tint of the color corrector on your skin would mix with your foundation and you would end up with a very strange shade of foundation. The premise is actually faulty from the beginning. I do not believe that pink skin needs to be more yellow and yellow skin needs to be more pink. All skin tones are equally fine and can be enhanced with the right makeup colors. There is no one skin color that is preferable over another. What a preposterous, narrow idea! The foundation, blush, eyeshadows, and lipstick colors are the best tools for enhancing or toning down your skin color without adding another layer makeup on your face.

How Much Makeup?

It is completely up to you how much makeup you choose to wear. There is no one application or design that is right for everyone. You do not "need" to wear a foundation or any other part of a makeup look if you don't want to. There are, however, very good reasons to use products that can improve your makeup look and I will explain these to you. The ultimate decision is up to you, depending on what makes you comfortable and whether or not you want to wear any makeup at all. There are also levels of makeup application that are more difficult or more formal, and I will address these too.

How do you decide for yourself how much makeup to use? As I said before, it depends on the image you want to project, what statement you want to make. For example, wearing a business suit instead of a jogging outfit to an office meeting makes a definite statement and it would make an even bigger statement if you were to do it the other way around. Because people react to the way we look and because makeup is a part of how we look, whether we like it or not, makeup reveals who we are. To be sure your look is saying what you want it to, remember the concept of balance as you decide what's right for you.

What exactly is balance when it comes to makeup application? Balance is the way several different products, colors, and textures work together to create one statement. Just as wearing a business suit to jog in is inappropriate, so is wearing a fully applied makeup look with a jogging outfit. Also contributing to a lack of balance in your image is having any one part of your makeup be more noticeable or stand out more than any other part. The art of a beautiful makeup application is the flow of color (eyeshadow, blush, and lipstick) and line (how the colors are placed and blended) from one area of the face to another. When the flow of color and line is balanced, the viewer's eye never rests on any particular aspect of the application. For example, if you line your eyes with black liner and do not balance it out with a strong lipstick color or interesting eyeshadow, shading the eyes will look overdone instead of attractive. The same is true if you wear a strong lip color and leave your eyes unshaded: it too looks out of balance.

As you read the following descriptions of makeup products and application techniques, evaluate what you are presently wearing or considering changing based on this notion of balance. It is what you are admiring most when you look at beautifully applied makeup on a model in a fashion magazine—the even flow of color over the face.

Note: *For specific product recommendations, please refer to* Don't Go to the Cosmetics Counter Without Me.

Highlighting

The first two steps in applying a complete makeup outfit are to reduce the darkness under the eye (as with a highlighter) and then apply a foundation to even out the skin. Once that is done, the eyeshadows and blushes can blend on smoothly over an even palette instead of varying degrees of skin textures and colors. Whether you start your application with the highlighter or the foundation depends more on personal preference than anything else and on the color of the highlighter you use. For the sake of organization, I'll start with the highlighter.

The use of a highlighter under the eye is to offset the natural shadows that occur because of the way the eye is set into the skull and to tone down the veins showing through the thin skin under the eye that make it look dark. The natural shadow that is created by the eye being set back into the skull is often compounded by the skin's tendency to be dark under the eye. The first thing you need, then, is a white or light flesh-tone highlighter.

The logic for using a white or light flesh-tone color is the same basic rule you learned in Art 101. When you need to make a can of paint a lighter color, you use white or a lighter color than you started with. Any other color, or the same color, or a darker color than the paint would defeat the purpose. Blue, yellow, or regular shades of skin tone, such as your foundation color, will not make the undereye area lighter. When shopping for an effective highlighter, look for a color that is several shades lighter than your foundation, or you will find yourself still staring at dark circles under your eyes.

The other consideration to keep in mind is that the highlighter is meant to blend with your foundation so that no edges or abrupt lines of demarcation can be seen. If you use a flesh-tone highlighter it is critical that it be the same basic color as your foundation, only lighter. That way you will be assured of having the foundation and highlighter blend together under the eye. If you choose a highlighter that is a very different color than your foundation, it will mix with the foundation (where they intersect under the eye) and you will simply end up with a third color, which will not necessarily be any lighter and will definitely be different.

The best way to choose which color highlighter to wear is by following these next few suggestions. If the area under the eye is very dark, a flesh-tone highlighter will work best. If the undereye is only slightly shadowed, use a touch of white highlighter blended over or under your foundation. Using white over extremely dark circle tends to make the skin under the eye look gray.

You would only use the white or light flesh-tone highlighter if the area under the eye isn't already light by itself. If your undereye area is naturally white, like a goggle effect, it may be necessary to apply a highlighter color that is slightly darker then the color of your foundation under the eye to reduce that masklike separation.

If you've decided to use a white highlighter, apply this highlighter first and then blend your foundation over it. The two mix together under the eye to create a highlighted effect. If you are using a flesh-tone highlighter, first apply your foundation all over your face, including under your eyes and on your eyelid, blending well, and then apply your highlighter, blending it over the undereye area.

There are times when I am wearing minimal makeup, for a more casual "Saturday" face, and I wear only highlighter and no foundation. If you want to lighten the undereye area when you are not wearing a foundation, choose a second foundation color or highlighter color that is only slightly lighter than your regular foundation. Or choose a highlighter that is a shade darker than the one you use with your foundation. I prefer using a lighter-colored foundation worn as a highlighter under the eye when I am not wearing foundation over the rest of my face, because it goes on thinner than most highlighters, giving sheerer coverage. This way the undereye area won't stand out as being the only area of my face that has makeup applied to it.

In the past it was almost impossible to find a good selection of highlighter colors. Now the tide has turned and some lines offer many (sometimes too many) shades to choose from. When shopping for a highlighter, the primary thing to look for is a shade that is lighter than your foundation, but not so light it sticks out, and a smooth texture to assure blending and staying power.

Types of Highlighters

Highlighters come in basically three different forms: sticks, creamy liquids or creams .

Stick Highlighters

Description: Stick highlighters come in tubes like lipsticks.

Application: They are applied to the undereye area much like a lipstick is applied to the mouth. They can be applied over or under your foundation, depending on how much coverage you want; under the foundation provides less coverage and over the foundation provides more. Dab the stick over the undereye in dots and then blend together. Avoid wiping it on like a matte streak of color. That tends to build up too much makeup, causing the highlighter to crease in the lines around the eye.

Pros: Depending on their consistency, stick highlighters can provide excellent coverage for very dark circles under the eye.

Cons: Oftentimes the texture of stick highlighters is rather dry and thick, which makes them difficult to blend without overpulling the skin under the eye. They also go on too heavily, which can create an obvious makeup look. Some stick highlighters can also be quite greasy, which can create a less obvious look, but can also slip too easily into the lines around the eyes.

Liquid Highlighters

Description: Liquid highlighters generally come in small squeeze-tube containers or long, thin tubes with wand applicators.

Application: Use your finger or the wand applicator to transfer the liquid highlighter in small dots of color under the eye area.

Pros: Depending on their consistency, liquid highlighters provide very light, even coverage.

Cons: Depending on their consistency, liquid highlighters have just the opposite problem of the stick highlighters: they can have too much movement and be hard to control. It is important when applying undereye highlighters to keep the color *just* under the eye. If the highlighter is too greasy or loose it can spread too easily, highlighting the cheek and parts of the face you don't want highlighted. Some liquid highlighters can go on too thin, offering very little coverage.

Cream Highlighters

Description: Cream highlighters come in a small pot and typically have a smooth, creamy, somewhat firm texture.

Application: Depending on their consistency, cream highlighters can go on easily with your fingertips or a cotton swab, placing the color in dots under the eye area.

Pros: Cream highlighters can have a very pleasing, creamy consistency, and they can also be rather thick and heavy. Depending on the consistency, they can go on well and provide even coverage.

Cons: If the cream highlighter is too thick or greasy, it can cake under the eye and crease into the lines.

Techniques in Applying Highlighters

Application Techniques

Regardless of the type of highlighter you use, the application remains the same. Dab the color on with either your fingertips, a cotton swab (which you dampen with water to control the cotton fuzzies), or a wand, and place the highlighter in a half-inch crescent from the corner of the eye called the tear drop (see diagram A) out to approximately one-third of the way under the eye. Avoid applying the highlighter all the way under the eye in a sweeping solid half circle. Smoothing a highlighter, particularly a white highlighter, all the way around the eye can create a goggle effect. Only apply the highlighter to the eyelid when it is also dark and could use some lightening.

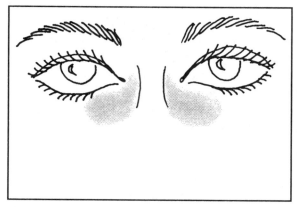

A) HIGHLIGHTER
Place white concealer on with the index finger or cotton swab hugging the inside corner of the undereye area.

Blending Techniques

If you are using the white highlighter, do not do any blending until the foundation is applied to the face. First, the white goes on as described above, and then the foundation directly over it. After the foundation is smoothed into place, the last area you blend is the white highlighter together with the foundation under the eye, dabbing while you blend. If you are using a flesh-tone highlighter, apply it in the same crescent shape described above *after* the foundation is blended evenly all over the face and eye area. Once the highlighter is in place over the foundation, carefully blend it out and under the eye in a dabbing motion, making sure you cannot see the edge where the highlighter stops and the foundation starts.

Regardless of the color highlighter you choose, always blend the foundation and highlighter together under the eye, being careful not to spread the highlighter onto the cheek or over the nose. The trick is to keep the highlighter blended only over the area where it is needed. As you may already know, highlighter is often recommended for use over facial lines to make them less apparent. For photography and stage that is a great technique; for every day it can create a heavier, more obvious look than is appropriate for daytime.

Highlighters can also be used over the central, flat part of the nose, the top of the cheekbone, the center of the chin, and the center of the forehead for accent and enhancement. These options tend to be complicated and time-consuming, even for women adept at applying their makeup, and most importantly, you can net the same results by applying the rest of your makeup correctly. I've used none of those techniques with my makeup as it appears on the cover of this book, and all those areas appear nicely highlighted because of the way I've applied the rest of my makeup. If you do choose to highlight these areas, place your highlighter in dots over your foundation in these areas and blend well, controlling the color so it does not spread all over your face.

Highlighter mistakes to avoid:

1 Do not wear a bright pink, orange, coral, or ash shade of highlighter.

2 If you can see the highlighter under your eye, you've chosen the wrong color.

3 Apply a moisturizer under the eye if the skin is dry to prevent the highlighter from caking.

4 Do not forget to blend the foundation and highlighter together so there are no hard edges.

5 Try the highlighter and wear it for a while before you buy it to be sure it doesn't crease into the lines around the eye.

6 Do not wear a highlighter that goes on thick or dry: it can cake under the eye and exaggerate wrinkles.

7 Do not wear a highlighter that is too greasy: it can crease in the lines and make them look more distinct.

Foundation

Personally, I've never been fond of the whole process of smearing foundation all over my face or even part of my face. I totally understand when women complain about feeling "made up" when they wear a foundation. So why do I recommend using foundation at all? Because of the even palette most foundations create on the skin. An even palette means the skin has a uniform color, texture, and appearance so that when you apply your blush and eyeshadows, the color looks even instead of choppy. *But at no time should the skin look like it has a layer of foundation on it!* If you are already blessed with a totally even complexion, then you will still want to consider wearing a foundation because of how it helps the other colors go on more evenly. If you try to blend blushes and eyeshadows without foundation, the likelihood is that they will go on choppy. Foundation is needed to keep those powdered colors in place. Since skin all by itself has no adhesive properties, foundation gives the rest of the makeup something to hold on to evenly. Blushes and eyeshadows have some ability to cling, but not much. They have more in common with baby powder then anything else. Ever put powder on after showering? Where does most of the powder end up? Right on the floor. Applying powder shadows and blushes can net a similar result if a foundation isn't there to prevent them from falling off.

Blending Techniques: The best tool to use when applying foundation is a flat, square, or round one-quarter-inch-thick sponge that doesn't have holes and is not made out of foam rubber. The shape and density of this kind of sponge provides the smoothest application possible. Cotton balls or cotton pads will deposit tiny pieces of themselves all over your face. Also, when you try to blend with a cotton ball, because of how well cotton absorbs, you end up wiping more foundation off than on. Fingers are also not a good choice to use when trying to blend foundation in place. Your fingers will streak and blend the makeup unevenly. Remember the streaky appearance finger painting creates on a piece of paper? Using your fingers on your face can have the same result.

The sponges that you frequently find for sale or in use at most cosmetics counters are the thick-wedged foam rubber sponges. These sponges are very difficult to use and I don't recommend them. They are not only hard to wash, they drag over the skin, which makes blending difficult. And because they're so thick, most of the foundation is absorbed into the sponge where you can't get to it, which can waste a lot of product. Wedge sponges are used for traditional theatrical makeup. They are great for applying grease stick or pancake foundations, which require more "pull" across the face in order to apply them evenly, but that is the last thing you need when wearing a water-based, lightweight foundation.

Natural sponges, which you rarely find anymore, have holes that will also cause problems when they're used for blending foundation. Because of their thickness, too much foundation is absorbed. Also, because these natural sponges aren't flat, it is almost impossible to get an even application. Imagine a paintbrush shaped like this.

To achieve an even application with your nice, flat, square sponge, shake some of the foundation from the bottle onto the sponge, then transfer the foundation to the face by dabbing the sponge over the skin. You can also use your fingers to transfer the foundation in dots from the bottle to the face and then use the sponge to blend the dots. Start by placing the foundation generously over the *central* area of the face, avoiding the sides of the face near the hairline, jaw, and chin. The foundation can go on in large patches or small dots all over the nose, eyelids, cheeks, and forehead, but only in this central area. At this stage, before you've started blending, avoid placing the foundation all over the face, which can cause too much foundation to be blended into the hairline and the jaw area, where you need the least amount of foundation to go (see diagram B).

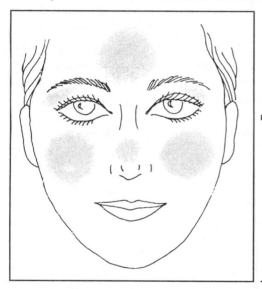

B) FOUNDATION

With a sponge, apply foundation generously to the central area of the face only, concentrating on the upper $\frac{2}{3}$. Then blend with a dry sponge in a down and outward motion. Always avoid placing color near the jaw. Over the eye, fold sponge in half and dab foundation in place.

Once the foundation is on the face, you can begin using your sponge to start blending the foundation evenly. Holding the sponge between your first three fingers and thumb, spread the foundation down and out over the entire face with a stroking, buffing motion in the direction of the hair. (Going against the direction of the hair growth on your face will coat the hair with too much foundation.) The idea is to blend the foundation color from the center of the face, where you initially placed it, into the perimeters of the face, leaving no line of demarcation at the jaw- or hairline. Use the edge of the sponge without foundation to dab or buff away any excess that tends to collect under the eye or around the nose. You can also use the sponge to wipe away any of the excess that gathers at the jaw- or hairline. When blending the foundation, do not try to force it into the skin. There is a fine line between blending something on and wiping something off. Instead, blend a thin layer over the face, smoothing it with your sponge as you go.

If you have not applied the highlighter before the foundation, you can now apply your highlighter and blend that into place. If you choose to use a white highlighter, follow the same procedure as above except first blend the foundation all over the face and leave the area under the eye for last. After you are done smoothing the foundation over the face, you are left with a few dots of foundation and a few dots of white highlighter waiting patiently under the eye. Now you blend the white highlighter together with the foundation under the eye by dabbing—not wiping— with the sponge.

If you choose to use a flesh-tone highlighter, you need to blend the foundation in place under the eye as well as over the rest of the face. The next step is to apply the flesh-tone highlighter over this area and then dab it into place with your finger or sponge. The white highlighter is blended together with the foundation. The flesh-tone highlighter is blended on over the foundation after the foundation has already been applied and blended.

Watch out for the jaw and neck. This is very important. Never ever put makeup of any kind on the neck; you do not want your makeup to end up on your collar. Also, your foundation should match your skin so exactly, and go on so sheer, that you only need to blend down to an inch or more above the jawline. This way you won't leave a line of demarcation at the jaw where the foundation stops and the neck begins.

Always double-check your blending. There are places on the face you will be likely to miss with foundation. These are the corners of the nose, the tip of the nose, the corners of the eyes (especially over the highlighter), and the edge along the lower eyelashes. There are also places that are likely to end up wearing foundation that shouldn't. These are the ears, the jawline, and the hairline, especially blond hairlines. Be careful to remove this foundation if you've gone past your mark. Both situations can make your makeup appear sloppy.

Never let your sponge get too far away. Your sponge is a wonderful blending tool you should keep near you at all times. When the edges of your blush or shadows need softening, you can work with the side of the sponge that was used to spread the foundation over the face to blend out the hard edges. Using the side of the sponge that has foundation on it as opposed to the dry edge allows the sponge to glide over the blush or eyeshadows without streaking it or rubbing it off.

Applying a Mini-application of Foundation

If you dislike the feel of foundation like I do or you want to wear the least amount of foundation possible, and yet you want the benefits that wearing a foundation provides, there is an alternative. The thing most women don't like about foundation is how it feels all over the face. One of the ways to solve that problem is to not wear foundation all over the face, because basically it isn't necessary. Remember, foundation is only needed to give the blush and eyeshadows something to adhere to. If the foundation color matches the face exactly—and after you finish this section it will—you can apply a mini-application of foundation over those areas where the blush and eye makeup will be placed. This way you won't feel heavily made up and the blush and eyeshadows will still go on evenly.

For a mini-application, place the foundation only over a mask-shaped area between the eyes and mouth, including the nose and cheeks. Coverage is not needed on the chin, forehead, or jaw area. Be sure to blend the edges carefully with your sponge. Apply the highlighter the same way you would for a full makeup application.

Finding the Perfect Foundation Color

I cannot stress this point enough; skin and foundation color should match exactly. If you are pale that's okay—accept the fact that you are pale and buy a light foundation that matches exactly. Do not buy a foundation that will make your face look a shade or two darker. Even with that slight a difference you run the risk of having a more obvious makeup application than you really want, particularly in daylight. The trick is to find a foundation that matches your skin perfectly and goes on sheer.

I wish choosing a foundation wasn't all that complicated, but it is. The crux of the problem is that when you're told to match the foundation with your skin tone, exactly what is meant by *skin tone*?

Traditional names associated with skin color are *olive*, when the skin appears ashen or green in color; *sallow*, when the skin has a yellow or golden shade; and *ruddy*, when the skin has overtones of pink or red. This is true for all women, including women of color. You may have been told that you are a particular "season" and your wardrobe *and* foundation color should be a specific undertone, either cool (blue tone) or warm (yellow tone). Unfortunately, this information can be misleading when it comes to choosing a foundation color (however, it is fine to use when choosing clothing colors).

If your skin color is ashen, are you going to choose an ashen foundation and look more green? Or if your face is very pink are you going to buy a pink foundation and look pink all over? Or if your face has cool undertones are you going to wear a blue tone foundation and look sickly? When purchasing a foundation, whether your skin color is olive, sallow, or ruddy, or your skin tone cool or warm, isn't what's important. What is important is to identify your exact flesh color and find a foundation that matches it, regardless of the underlying color or tone. For the most part, regardless of race, nationality, or age, your foundation, 99 percent of the time, should be some shade of neutral beige, tan, or dark brown and a hundred shades in between without any orange, pink, green, or blue color in it.

Specifically, your foundation color is always going to be some degree of palest neutral beige (with no orange, pink, green or blue color), to tan (with no orange or green color), to the darkest chocolate brown (with no orange or green color). I know this might sound a bit confusing. But when you think about it, you haven't really seen any pink, orange, green, blue or ashen people. Foundations that are these colors are simply the worst you can buy. Please refer to *Don't Go to the Cosmetics Counter Without Me* for specific foundation recommendations. This will help you avoid the wrong foundation colors.

There are a few exceptions to this rule. Native American women, a small percentage of African-American women, and some Polynesian women do indeed have a red cast to their skin and in those instances this information should be ignored. Because they have a slight red cast to their skin color, they need to look for foundations that have a slight reddish cast to them, but that's only a hint of red and not orange. Everyone needs to avoid orange shades of makeup and there are a lot of them out there.

Question: If all the fashion magazines and makeup experts talk about foundations being sheer and matching the skin exactly, how come so many women I see of all ages are wearing heavy-looking, obvious foundations? Some of it is this confusion about skin tone and foundation color I've been talking about; some of it is not checking your foundation in the daylight; and some of it is that many women hate their skin. Rather than arguing the emotional ramifications of disliking your skin, because I probably can't talk you out of it, let me just say that covering your face in an obvious layer of foundation is not the way to take care of it. That only makes matters worse. It is essential to an attractive makeup application of any kind to start with a good, sheer foundation. Even if you feel you are in need of a foundation that provides good coverage, coverage that shows is a monumental mistake and can negatively affect the entire makeup application.

What Is Skin Tone?

Skin tone is the underlying color of the skin. What generates skin tone? For those women with *ruddy* skin tone, the skin's pink appearance comes from the tiny capillaries found close to the surface of the skin. How apparent the pinkness is depends on circulation, the thickness of the skin, and the amount of melanin present in the skin. A pink-looking skin can also come from broken capillaries that look like tiny red lines on the face, sunburn, skin irritation, or acne. *Sallow* describes skin that has little to no pinkness present and in which the strong, natural yellow-brown tone of the skin is predominant. *Olive* skin is similar to sallow skin except there is a good deal of melanin present. For African-American skin color the gold in the skin is oftentimes fairly obvious. Sometimes women of color can have problems with the skin color becoming ashen or gray as the skin matures. The exact reason for this is not known, although it could be the result of the skin becoming thicker as it ages.

For Caucasian and some Asian women there is a skin color that is often referred to as *porcelain*. This indicates an even, light, pale complexion that is not ruddy, sallow, or olive. This skin tone is the one you see most often on the covers of fashion magazines. There is definitely a strong desire in Western culture to recreate this porcelain skin tone. There is also a great deal of emphasis placed on a tanned skin color, which is also often depicted in fashion magazines. For many women, particularly older women, there is a strong desire to recreate a blushing pink, youthful appearance. All of these are impossible to reproduce without looking unnatural and made up. The thought of buying a pink, rose, or orange-toned foundation may seem like you would be smoothing on pink, rosy, glowing skin, but believe me, that is not the case. All you will be putting on is a foundation that will look very phony on your skin and that is difficult to blend.

The foundation is only the base that you then build the color design upon, and because of that it is essential for it to be neutral (or as neutral as possible) and not rose, pink, orange, or green. The "color" on the face is added to selected areas when you apply the blush, eyeshadows, and lipstick—and not all over the face with your foundation. Choose a realistic foundation color that might not sound pretty but will certainly give you the best results.

This same rule holds true for women of color. Their skin needs to be matched with a golden shade of brown, chocolate, or ebony foundation that should have not be orange or ashen. The names of darker-colored foundations always sound beautiful, so you will need to be extra careful not to be seduced into buying them if they do not match your own skin color. In fact, dark-colored foundations tend to be orange in color sometimes more than lighter ones. A foundation called Cinnamon might sound good, but you could be painting red tones on your skin when what you want is golden brown or golden black.

An Exception to the Rule

Although in theory you are attempting to match the skin color of your face exactly when you choose a foundation, there are those women who need to be more concerned about the color of their neck. In some cases it is more important to match the foundation to the color of the neck than to the face. If the face is darker than the neck and you put on a foundation that matches the face, it will look like a mask because of the difference in color between the two. The opposite is also true. If the face is lighter than the neck and you put on a foundation that matches the face, it will still look like a mask because of the difference in color between these two areas. This color difference doesn't happen often, but it happens often enough so that some of you should know about it. In this situation match the foundation more to the neck color or to a color in between the neck and the face color. To make sure it is the right color, try it on and check it in the daylight for a natural appearance.

The Final Decision

Regardless of how you finally decide to go about choosing a foundation color, there is absolutely only one way to be sure the foundation is right for you: apply the color all over the face and check it outside in the daylight. Check it from all angles and then decide if it matches your skin exactly. If it was carefully applied and there are any lines of demarcation at the jaw area, or if it appears too thick or too greasy, or if it gives the face an orange or pinkish tint, or if it looks too heavy and opaque instead of sheer and light, you will need to go back to the testers. In fact, you may need to test several types before you've found the right foundation.

A popular technique for narrowing down your choice before you apply one specific foundation all over the face is to test several different colors that look like good possibilities on the face first by placing them in stripes in a row over the cheek area. The best choice will be the one that blends almost perfectly with your skin color. The wrong choices will stick out with hard edges that don't disappear into your skin.

The best of all worlds would be to wait at least two hours after you've applied the foundation and then check it again in the daylight. How a foundation wears during the day—does it change color or become too greasy or dry as the day passes?—can only be evaluated after wearing it for a while. Once you've assessed all these details in the daylight, you can safely make a final determination as to whether this is the right color or type of foundation for you. If at all possible, please take the time to follow this procedure. It is the only guarantee you can have of finding the right foundation. My advice will lead you in the right direction, but if you let the salesperson or the lighting at the cosmetics counters be your only source of information, it will be pure luck if you end up with the right color.

Types of Foundation

Now that you know how to apply your foundation and which color foundation you need to buy, the last stone to look under is what *type* of foundation is best suited to your skin. There are four basic types of foundation available at the cosmetics counters: oil-free, water-based, oil-based, and the new powder-based foundations.

Oil-free Foundation

Description: Oil-free foundation has no oil of any kind in it. There are three forms this foundation comes in. One looks like a bottle of colored water that contains mostly talc, alcohol, and coloring agents; another looks like a traditional creamy, thick foundation that contains water, waxes, emulsifiers, and coloring agents; and the last is mostly glycerin with the coloring ingredients and waxes comprising the other part.

Application: Oil-free makeup that is creamy in texture, rather than watery, goes on like most other foundations. The differences appear after it is blended and dries quickly into place with a matte finish that shows no reflection or shine. The alcohol-based oil-free foundation is more difficult to apply because it is so watery that it may not give much coverage at all, and it tends to run and streak as you apply it, even with a sponge, and can look powdery. Glycerin-based foundations are unique in that they are more like a liquid than a cream, but they give better coverage than the alcohol-based foundations.

Pros: The creamy oil-free foundation is the best foundation choice for those women who do not want their skin to shine at all, want even coverage, and like a matte look. This is the type of foundation I wear for television appearances. It will also last much longer on oily skin than any other foundation type, which for some women is a very desirable, if not essential, effect.

Cons: The disadvantage of using the cream-type oil-free foundation is that some of them can go on rather heavy and masklike, leaving the skin feeling quite dry and taut. In order to get this makeup on evenly, it is best to blend quickly or it will dry in place before you know it, and then it is difficult to blend further. You have to get it on right the first time, because once it's on it doesn't move easily. In terms of applying eyeshadow and blush, this foundation can be hard to work over. Because oil-free makeup has less movement than foundations that contain a small amount of oil (such as water-based foundations), the powders you use will have a tendency to stick to it, which can make blending and correcting mistakes a bit irksome.

I never recommend the alcohol-based foundations because of their poor coverage and the irritation alcohol can cause the skin. Glycerin-based oil-free foundation is an option, but it is not my preference. When glycerin is such a large percentage of a product, as it is with these foundations, it can prove to be irritating to the skin. I also find these foundations tricky to use—hard to blend, and often the color tends to shift after you've worn it for a while. But for those women who can work with it and don't have problems with the color changing or irritation, it may be an interesting option.

Women of color or women with tanned skin should avoid as much as possible using an oil-free foundation, even if it is the right color, because it can look gray and ashen after it is applied to the face and dries. Skin that shows no shine or reflection in general tends to look dull gray with this kind of foundation and that becomes even more true for women of color. The major reason, if not the only reason, to choose an oil-free foundation is to avoid adding any more shine to the face than the skin has created on its own.

Water-based Foundation

Description: *Water-based* does not mean *oil-free*; it simply means that the first ingredient is water and the second or third ingredient is oil. These foundations look like a somewhat thick liquid and pour slowly out of the bottle.

Application: A water-based foundation, if applied correctly, should feel lightweight. In most cases it can go on in an even, thin layer. If you want heavy coverage you will probably be disappointed in a water-based foundation.

Pros: Most water-based foundations are best for those with normal to dry skin. It is the perfect type to wear without the aid of a moisturizer for these skin types, but it is also fine to wear with a moisturizer if your skin needs it. The oil part of this foundation gives it good movement, which makes blending a pleasure and allows blushes and eyeshadows to blend on effortlessly and evenly over the face. Mistakes are easily buffed away with the sponge.

Cons: If you have oily skin you will almost always be better off and prefer an oil-free foundation over the water-based type. The little bit of oil in a water-based foundation will show shine almost immediately if you have oily skin. Those of you who do not have oily skin but have a paranoia about any shine on the face will not like the effects of a water-based foundation; the small amount of oil in this cosmetic may make you nervous. For the most part, I personally don't feel there are any disadvantages to using water-based foundations and I recommend them wholeheartedly. Water-based foundation is also a great option for women of color. The slight amount of oil it contains helps create a nice glow on the skin, preventing darker skin tones from appearing dull or ashen.

If you are concerned with the small amount of shine water-based foundations leave behind on the skin, try adding a light dusting of loose powder. You can apply the powder all over the face after you've blended the foundation in place to reduce the shine.

Oil-based Foundation

Description: Oil-based foundations have oil as their first ingredient and water usually as their second or third ingredient. Oil-based foundations feel greasy and thick, look greasy and thick, and go on greasy, but not necessarily thick. You can blend an oil-based foundation to a very thin, sheer layer of makeup.

Application: Because of the tendency of oil-based foundations to be thick, you can help blend a thinner layer of foundation over the face by adding water to the sponge before you begin blending. If you wear face powder over this type of foundation the oil will grab the talc and the face can appear coated and heavily made up even if you blend it on thin. The same is true for blushes and eyeshadows—they will go on heavier because of the increased oil on the skin, and they will also become darker once applied.

Pros: Oil-based foundations can be very good for women with extremely dry skin.

Cons: Oil-based foundations are very greasy, thick, and heavy, and tend to look that way on the skin unless you are very adept at blending. They also have a tendency to turn orange on the skin because of the way the extra oil affects the pigment in the foundation. The same can be true for women of color, and including those with dark tans. Oil-based foundations can look orange after they are worn for a while. The typical recommendation for using oil-based foundations is to add water to your sponge so that it goes on thinner, more like a water-based foundation. But that can be tricky to gauge and can cause the makeup to streak. Why not just use a water-based foundation in the first place and skip the negatives of the oil-based foundation?

Powder-based Foundation

Description: These foundations are relatively new on the cosmetic scene. They come in a compact and look like a pressed powder. This is a unique product because almost all of them have a wonderful creamy, silky feel, but when applied to the skin, they blend on more like a powder.

Application: You can apply these foundations only with a sponge. This is the easiest way to get the smoothest application. Don't worry about the powder looking flaky like loose or pressed powder can. These foundations go on smoothly and evenly as good foundations should.

Pros: Powder-based foundations are great for women with normal to oily skin. They blend on easily and quickly, last all day, don't change color, and feel wonderful on the skin.

Cons:The only negative to wearing powder-based foundation is for those women with dry skin. This is not a good option if you have any amount of flaky skin, regardless of your skin type. Because of its powder content, this foundation can be too drying for someone with dry skin and because of the way it goes on it can make the skin look more dry and flaky.

Foundation mistakes to avoid:

1 Do not wear pink, coral, orange, or ash-colored foundation.

2 Do not use your fingers to blend your foundation over the face.

3 Do not wear foundation unless it matches your skin color as much as possible.

4 Do not wear a foundation that is lighter than your skin, or you will end up looking chalky or pale.

5 Do not apply a thick layer of foundation. *Thin* and *sheer* are the operative words when it comes to applying foundation.

6 Do not buy a foundation before trying it on and checking it in the daylight.

7 Do not wear oil-based foundations unless you have very, very dry skin. Oil-based foundations can look greasy and appear more orange and pink than other types of foundation.

8 Do not wear oil-free foundations unless you have very oily skin. Oil-free foundations can look quite thick and matte and make lines on the face more evident.

9 Do not buy foundations that you haven't tried on and checked out in the daylight.

Brushes

Before we can go on to powders, eyeshadows, and blushes, it is crucial to discuss your most important makeup applicator and blending tool after the sponge, and that is the brush. I recommend brushes when applying powders of any kind because they are simply the best way to apply these. You would be hard put to find a makeup artist anywhere who disagrees with this one. Don't use those little doll-size applicators or sponge-tip sticks that come with eyeshadows and blushes. Use good, full-size, thick-haired, soft bristle brushes to help assure even application of your contour, blush, and eye makeup. This is as good a time as any for you to throw away those little brushes that come packed with the compacts, which are too small to match the size of anyone's cheek or eye.

The two rules to follow when choosing the right brush are 1) The brush should match the size of the area it is to be used on, and 2) Brushes should not be so stiff that they scratch the face nor so soft as to be floppy and difficult to control. A good brush makes all the difference between a quick, smooth makeup job and a sloppy, streaky, time-consuming make-up struggle.

For the most part brushes are foolproof tools for applying makeup, but sometimes it is possible to use brushes incorrectly. I've seen enough women use their brushes in a rubbing or wiping motion on the face to know how often it can happen. Many women beat at their faces with a wild brushing motion as they attempt to apply their blush and eyeshadows. There truly is an easier way. Do not rapidly wipe, beat, or rub the brush against the face. Inadvertently, you may be removing what you just put on, not to mention the foundation underneath. Do brush in short, purposeful motions that glide over the skin.

Whenever there is a distinct line where the brushstroke was placed or you feel an urge to use your hand to blend what you've just applied, you are most likely not using the brush properly or your brush is too stiff for a soft application. (You may also have applied your foundation too thickly or used too greasy a foundation, which means you need to read over the foundation section again.) You should not be blending anything with your fingers—only with your brush or the flat, square, thin sponge you used to apply your foundation. Remember, your sponge is for applying foundation and softening edges of your blush, contour, and eyeshadows. Do not apply blush with a sponge.

Something else that is critical to using brushes effectively—even though it may seem insignificant at first—is the way you pick up the powder on your brush before you apply it. Never smash or rub your brush into the powder. Rather, place your brush into the powder gently, without moving the bristles. You don't want to see the brush hair bend or splay (see diagram C). Always stroke through the powder evenly and be sure to knock the excess powder off the brush before you apply it to the face. This prevents applying too much color to the first place your brush touches on the face.

A wise investment for any makeup case is good brushes. Always feel the brush to be sure you are buying a soft but firm one. Bristles that are too loose or too stiff will be hard to use. Even though I want you to buy a good set of brushes, I do not recommend you buy a packaged set of brushes. More often than not you end up getting brushes you will never use. It is best to find a store that sells brushes individually (most major department stores do nowadays) and to select from these the ones you want. Depending on how complicated a makeup design you wear the maximum number of brushes you need are three basic eyeshadow brushes, one large square-shaped brush (sometimes called a No. 10) and two round medium-size brushes (often called fluff brushes), an eyeliner brush (sometimes called a 00 brush), a blush brush, a contour brush, a large powder brush, a brow and lash brush, and a lip brush. I will discuss which brushes to use where and how as we go through each makeup step.

Brush mistakes to avoid:

1 Do not forget to knock the excess powder off the brush before you apply the color to your face.

2 Do not use hard or stiff brushes.

3 Do not wipe or rub the brush across the face. Gently brush the color on in short strokes.

4 Do not use brushes that are too soft or if the bristles are too sparse.

C) Proper Use of Brushes

Eyeliner

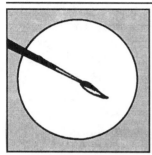

DO
Use the
flat side of
the brush

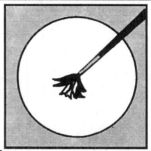

DO NOT
Use the tip.
Do not
splay the
brush

Eyeshadow

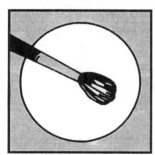

DO
Use the
flat edge of
the brush

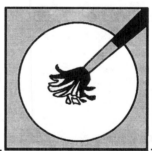

DO NOT
Splay the
brush

Blush, Powder or Contour

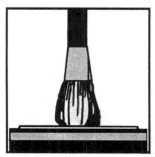

DO
Use the full
head of the
brush

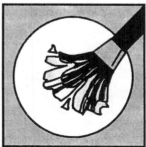

DO NOT
Splay the
brush

5 Do not forget to use your sponge to blend out hard edges and soften your color application.

Powdering

This is another one of those areas where my opinion takes a departure from the mainstream. I believe it is not necessary to powder immediately after applying your foundation, regardless of the foundation. The less powder you build up on your face, the less made up you will look. Also, I am convinced that a matte foundation (unless you have oily skin) makes the face look dull. Some amount of shine to the face is very attractive. I think it is a 1950s notion that the face should not shine at all and that a woman must constantly wipe powder over her face to reduce the shine. After a foundation is applied, the slight shine that is left behind (except with oil-free foundation) gives the face a wonderful glow. The advice you will get at the cosmetics counters is to apply your foundation and then immediately apply your powder. But then, of course, salespeople are quick to sell you shiny blush, shiny eyeshadows, and shiny lipsticks so your cheeks, lips, and eyes shine but not your face. I think that is backward thinking. Powder is fine to use for touch-ups as the day goes by to dust down excessive shine, but to start out wearing it can be a mistake.

Description: Powdering the face after applying your foundation is definitely optional and depends in the final analysis on your own personal preference. The need for powder is based on the amount of shine you want to reduce after you apply your makeup or as the day goes by.

Application: When you powder your face it is probably best to use loose, translucent powder instead of pressed powder to achieve the sheerest look. Pressed powder is heavier than loose powder, but pressed powder is more convenient and less messy. Whichever works best for you is fine. What is essential, though, is to choose a powder that is the same color as your foundation. If you choose a shade of powder that is lighter than your foundation it can end up making you look pasty and pale, and a darker one can make you look like you're wearing a mask.

Apply the powder with a large, full, round brush. Avoid using a sponge or powder puff, which can pack too much powder onto the face. Pick up some of the powder on the full of the brush, knock out the excess, and brush it on in the same motion and direction you did the foundation. That will keep everything going in the same direction and help retain a smooth appearance. Before powdering, use your sponge or a facial tissue to dab away excess oil from the face.

Pros: Powdering the face is an effective way to handle the oil shine that can make the skin look slippery and greasy.

Cons: There are really no negatives to wearing powder, except overdoing it and building up too much powder on the skin or choosing the wrong color. Other than that, powdering is a basic step to keeping makeup looking fresh during the day.

Powdering mistakes to avoid:

1 Do not apply more than the sheerest layer necessary to take away excess shine. The face can handle only so much powder before it starts looking thick and heavy.

2 Do not powder more than necessary during the day. Powder the face only once or twice a day to prevent buildup.

3 Do not forget to dab off excess oil from the face before you apply your powder to help prevent buildup.

4 Never powder the face with a color that is lighter or darker than your foundation. Powder should match your foundation color exactly.

5 Never powder your face with a white, orange, pink, or coral shade of powder. It will make you look either pale or overly made up.

6 Do not buy powder without testing it over your foundation before you buy it. The color of your powder is as important as your foundation color.

Contouring

Although contouring is most definitely an optional step for most daytime makeup applications, it is still rather intriguing and worthwhile to most women. Contouring the face is the art of creating or increasing shadows in certain areas so the face appears to have more structure and definition. It involves using brown tones of blush to contour along the sides of the nose, at the sides of the forehead, under the cheekbone, and in the center of the chin to add color, definition, and shape to the face.

For the most part, the art of contouring to reshape the face has somewhat died down. The likely reason for its recent demise is that believable-looking contouring is difficult to master. Contouring takes skill and patience, which is more than most women have time to deal with every morning. Even if you decide to take the time, the frequent result is that a stripe of brown powder appears under the blush and that is not the way contouring is supposed to look. My strong recommendation is to think twice before incorporating this step into your daily makeup routine before you've practiced and developed the skill to apply this look softly.

Contouring is always done as a separate step with a completely different brush and color of powder than that of the blush application. Pinks, reds, and oranges are used in blushing; only brown colors are used in contouring. The safest contour shade to use if you have fair to medium-dark skin tones is one that looks like your skin color when it is tanned. A soft or rich golden shade of brown is generally the perfect color to use when trying to produce realistic shadows on the face. Shades of gray-brown can look dirty and shades of red-brown and mauve-brown can look like bruising on women with fair to medium-dark skin tones.

For women of color, particularly African-American women, either an extremely dark shade of golden brown or an ashy deep-brown color will work exceptionally well.

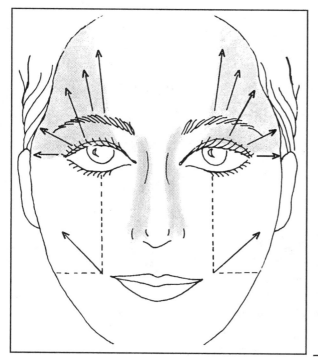

D) **CONTOURING**
Soften hard edges with your sponge. For temple contour reapply if needed to soften eyeshadow. Under cheekbone and nose contouring is optional.

Here are some rules of placement to help you most effectively contour your face (see diagram D).

Under or along the jawline. Avoid contouring or shading along any portion of the jawline. After you've gone through all the trouble to find a foundation that leaves no line of demarcation at the jaw, it does not make sense to add a brown stripe there and hope people believe it looks like a natural shadow. For pictures or possibly evening it can be passable, but it needs to be applied very carefully. Be careful! Shading under the jawline can also mean you will end up shading your collar at the same time.

Under the cheekbone. To find this area you will need two thin pencils, diagram D, and a well-lighted mirror. (You always need a well-lighted mirror when doing your makeup.) Take one of the pencils and place it vertically against your face, in alignment with the pupil, down along the cheek. Holding that in place, take the other pencil and place it horizontally against your face, parallel with your mouth, from the corner of the lips to the earlobe. Where these two pencils intersect is where the placement of your contour begins. This intersection should be approximately one-quarter inch behind your laugh line.

Place the center of your brush at this point and stroke the color straight back, aiming toward the middle of the ear. You will find that following these directions will put the color under your cheekbone. The area of application should be approximately a half inch in width with no definite edges visible. Use your sponge to soften hard edges.

The starting point for under-cheekbone contouring is almost always the same because the cheekbone corresponds nicely to the eye socket and the jawline. The end point at the ear, though, can be varied according to the effect you desire. The steeper the angle going toward the top of the ear, the longer the face will appear. If you have a square-shaped or round face, you might want to try contouring with a steeper angle. The longer the face (as an oblong or triangular face might be), the more straight back toward the middle of the ear the line can be. This, in effect, de-emphasizes the length of the face.

The contour brush I recommend is the one usually labeled for blush or rouge. This traditional blush brush is really too small for most cheeks, so it becomes a poor choice for blush application. The brush labeled for contouring is a poor choice for applying contour because it is usually too hard and flat and can make visible edges when you apply your color. When contouring, use the full of the blush brush. Knocking off the excess powder before applying and brushing in short, quick motions going back to the ear should net the best results.

Caution: *When applying the under-cheekbone contour, be sure never to blend or place the contour color below the mouth area, below the middle of the ear, or onto the cheekbone itself. There is also no need to suck in the sides of your mouth to help find your cheekbone—that will only help you find the sides of the mouth, not the cheekbone.*

The sides of the nose. The goal with this step, besides making the nose look narrower or longer, is to make the contour color look absolutely as soft as possible. The challenge of making this shading step look blended is that you have to restrict the color to the sides of the nose. You never want to accidentally blend the color of the nose contour onto the area under your eyes or on your cheeks. Take extra care to blend only a small amount of contour color on such an obvious focal point of the face.

The best technique for applying the nose contour is to take the brush you are using for contour and place the brush itself between your fingers and thumb, so the brush tip becomes somewhat flattened. This way the brush tip can more easily follow along the sides of your nose. Now, with your other hand, use your index finger and place it flat, down the center of the nose, take your contour brush and apply the contour color along the side of your finger. Where the brush falls against your finger is the area to be contoured. Once you've done this, remove your finger and softly apply the contour fully around the tip of the nose and on the flare of the nostrils. Following diagram D, continue the contour in a narrow, soft line up under the eyebrow, avoiding the corner of the eye and the center area between the eyebrows. This end point under the eyebrow will be an overlap spot for when you start applying your eyeshadow to hide any hard edges where the contour color stops. Another option for applying the nose contour is to use a very large, flat eyeshadow brush.

Although most women think that contouring the nose is strictly to make it look smaller or narrower, there is actually a more artistic reason for using this shading technique. If you're applying a full makeup, particularly for evening, and the nose is ignored, you will have color everywhere on your face except for a blank spot in the center of the face. Contouring the nose helps to achieve color balance for the rest of the face when you choose to wear a formal, full makeup application.

The temple area. Temple contour is a traditional step in makeup that is as basic as applying blush. The difference is that most women just don't know about it. Take a look at the cover of any fashion magazine and you will notice that most of the models have this contour applied. Temple contour creates a shade of color for the eyeshadow applied to the back of the eye area to blend into. When temple contour is neatly applied, the eyeshadow at the back of the eye doesn't end abruptly as a harsh-colored edge on a flesh-colored space. Without temple contour the forehead becomes a great bare wall against the color background of the cheeks and eyes.

The temple contour is placed at the back third of the under-eyebrow bone, directly out and up onto the forehead like a pie wedge without the edges. There are two ways to apply temple contour: either before the eyeshadows are applied or after the eye design is in place. If you apply the contour after the eye design, it is important to place the brush directly over the eyeshadows at the back third of the eye and then brush the contour all the way back to the hairline, about two inches wide at its fullest point (see diagram D). If you do the contour first, it is applied in the exact same place and in the same way, but when the eyeshadows are applied they blend directly over and onto the temple contour. Either way, the contour softens the back edge of the eyeshadows.

There are three common mistakes that can make temple shading look bad. The first is forgetting that this step begins at the *back* third of the under-eyebrow, brushing right on top of and over the back third of the entire eye area. The second is not brushing the contour directly over the eyebrow itself. If you try to avoid the eyebrow, you can make the application look choppy instead of smooth and even. The last is applying the color in a straight one-inch strip next to the eye instead of a softly blended two-inch pie wedge that is partially blended onto the forehead. Temple contour is a shaded area like the blush area, and it should never look like a stripe.

Contour mistakes to avoid:

1 Do not use a blush color to contour any part of your face. Only contour with a golden brown, red-brown, or chocolate-brown shade of contour.

2 Do not forget to blend hard edges. Contour should always look soft.

3 Do not use contour under the jaw or chin area during the day. It will look too obvious and possibly get on clothing.

4 Do not apply nose contour until you get used to blending it on softly. Nose contour can be tricky. It should never look like stripes down the sides of the nose.

Blush

Blushing is one of those parts of makeup application many women take for granted. The comment I hear most often is, "I've been doing that for years. I know how to put on blush." Yet it is so easy to make mistakes with this one and I see it all the time. Blush is one of the more prominent parts of any makeup routine, so when you do make a mistake—such as applying it too close to the lines around the eye, applying it like a stripe of color across the cheek, or applying the wrong color—it is very noticeable. I urge you to take time to learn how to apply blush properly.

I can't say that everyone agrees exactly where you are supposed to place your blush. There are many opinions on where it should start, where it should end, and how high or low to place it along the cheekbone. My strong opinion—and one I believe is held by most makeup artists—is to keep the blush on the cheekbone away from the eye area, making certain to blend the color under the cheekbone and starting the color about half an inch behind the laugh line. You might have been told by some makeup "experts" to start the blush no farther into the center of the face than the center of the eye. That can make the blush look very strange. Too far back, and you have missed a good portion of the cheekbone. The idea is to blush the entire cheekbone.

The best way to find the area to be blushed is almost the same as for contouring under the cheekbone. Using this method can be a fail-safe way to apply blush. Again, start with your two pencils and a well-lighted mirror. Place one of the pencils vertically against your face in alignment with the pupil along the center of the cheek. Place the other pencil horizontally at the underside of the nose, parallel with the mouth, from the nose to the center of the ear. At the intersection of these two pencils—down from the pupil and across from the *tip* of the nose—is where you begin your blush. This area will be approximately one-quarter to one-half inch behind the laugh line. Place the full of your brush here and then brush downward, being careful not to place any color below the level of the mouth, and moving back toward the center of your ear (see diagram E).

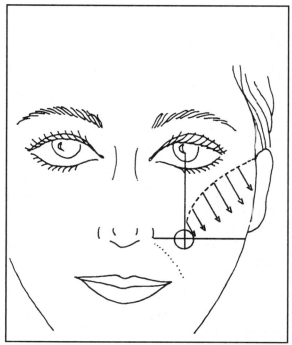

E) BLUSH PLACEMENT

Brush down and proceed back to ear. Do not blush by laugh lines or below mouth

Note: *Applying your blush by brushing down as opposed to back and forth will eliminate a stripe effect. The blush area should be about two inches thick with no hard edges. Always use your sponge to soften edges.*

Basically the most typical blush available is a compact powder. These are an excellent choice for all skin types. What about powder-based blushes? There are many of these now on the market and they are definitely an alternative to consider. They are best for women with normal to oily skin, because they can look too powdery on women with dry skin. These powder-based blushes go on easily, blend beautifully and come in great colors. Most powder-based blushes can be applied with either a brush or a sponge, although I prefer using a brush. Whichever is easiest for you and creates the softest look will be the best choice for you.

What about liquid or gel blushes? These are not my favorites and I would recommend strongly staying away from them. Liquid or gel blushes sound good when the salesperson is explaining them, but they just don't perform reliably. Both liquid and gel blushes can be very awkward to blend evenly, they tend to stain the cheek (which means they can flake off during the day), they can stain the pore (making the face look dotted with color), and they don't work well over foundation. If you have flawless skin and want to try a liquid or gel blush when you aren't wearing a foundation, give it a try, but don't buy anything until you check it out in the daylight and see how it wears during the day.

How much color is too much or too little? That is not an easy question to answer. Over the past two years pale blush has been in, but that is probably best for a trendy look, as opposed to a classic one. For most women a pale blush will look ghostly and pale. It is probably best to go softer than vivid when it comes to cheek color, but some color is definitely desirable and ultimately more attractive.

Blush mistakes to avoid:

1 Never blush close to the lines around the eye, as it makes them look more evident, as well as red and irritated.

2 Do not blush below the mouth or the laugh lines. Blush is only for the cheekbone.

3 Do not blush your nose, forehead, hairline, or chin. It can make the face look overly pink or red or made up.

4 Do not forget to use your sponge to blend out hard edges or smudges of blush. Blush should always be well blended, with no visible edges where the blush starts and stops.

If you are applying both blush and under-cheekbone contour, apply the contour color first and then blend the blush on top of and gradually down into the contour color. Then, using your sponge, blend until you meld the colors together into an attractive design. The trademark of an attractive design is not being able to see where one color stops and the other starts.

Eyeshadow

I've developed an eyeshadow application sequence that can help you build the eye design of your choice in either one, two, three, four, or five steps. The five steps are applied in a sequence of colors going from very light to gradually darker. Each color corresponds to a specific area of the eye. The basic technique is to apply the lighter color all over the entire eye area and then place each progressively darker shade in a more specific section of the eye area. To get through this sequence, let's start with how to use eyeshadow brushes, go on to how to choose where to place light and dark colors, and then talk about how to apply the design. Be sure to use diagram F for the terms used in the eyeshadow application descriptions. If any of the following descriptions are to make any sense at all, the diagrams must be referred to frequently for both information about placement and definition of terms.

Using brushes. Eyeshadow, as far as application technique goes, is applied exclusively with brushes. It is best to use brushes that are designed specifically for eyeshadow. Never use sponge-tip applicators; they drag across the eye and tend to blend colors in streaks. How you use the brush can make a vast difference in your blending technique and how smooth your eye design looks. I suggested before that when you apply contour or blush color it is best to use the full of the brush instead of the flat edge of the brush. When applying eyeshadow you do just the opposite and use the flat side of the brush. Gently wipe the brush through the eyeshadow, knock the excess off the brush, and apply it with long stroking motions. This motion of laying strips of color over the eye that overlap and blend together is the way to achieve an even, well-blended design.

It is important to always remember that the size of the brush should match the size of the eye area you are working on. If you have a large eye area, use a brush that is wide and full. If your eyelid is small, the brush should be smaller in width. Brushes that match the job are essential to getting makeup on effectively and efficiently. Be certain you are not using or purchasing brushes that have hard, coarse bristles, or you will end up with hard edges where your eyeshadow couldn't be blended, not to mention irritated skin.

Designing the Eye

Makeup books and cosmetics salespeople describe and demonstrate all kinds of eye designs—a dab of yellow in the center of the lid, teal across the crease, taupe above the teal, pink above the teal, and gray in the back corner of the lid. Not only do I think those designs are too complicated, I've never seen them on a model on the cover of any fashion magazine. In fact, even the makeup books and cosmetics lines that sell these pastel color sets rarely use them on their models. Although, Lancôme, Estée Lauder, Elizabeth Arden, Max Factor, Borghese, and most makeup lines sell vivid eyeshadows, the models in their ads rarely have them on.

The most beautiful makeup applications, the ones you admire the most on models and actresses, are neutral in color, not colorful. You can check this one out for yourself by looking at any fashion magazine. You're not going to see pastel eyeshadows applied to these faces. Too many competing colors over the eye area make the eye design distracting, and colors that are highly contrasting are hard to blend together. On the other hand, there is also a problem with designs that are too simple. Painting one color of eyeshadow across the lid—such as a bright blue, bright pink, or bright green—is also distracting, too colorful, and unfashionable.

The purpose of eyeshadows is to shape the eye, not color it. The only way to shape the eye is by shading it with neutral shades such as taupe, brown, gray, ash, beige, tan, mahogany, redwood, sable, charcoal, and black. The list of neutral colors and shades available is actually quite extensive. Color on the eyelid is best kept as subtle as possible, or you will end up creating an eye design that is more noticeable than your eye. The color on the face is provided by the lips and blush. More color on the eye can be overkill.

Be cautious about thinking you need to choose a design based on the need to correct a so-called problem, such as your eyes being too close together, too far apart, too round, or not round enough. There are no standard facial dimensions that define how attractive you or your eyes are.

The best way to choose which design to wear is by what image you want to project. The more shading you use, the more dramatic and formal the eye design becomes; the less shading, the more subtle and casual the design will appear. Another consideration for choosing one eye design over another is your ability and skill at applying makeup, personal preference, and time considerations. For example, if you are new or unaccustomed to wearing makeup, keep your entire makeup look simple until you become adept at the different application techniques. Also, if you have only a few minutes in the morning to get your makeup on, it is probably best to keep your routine simple. Trying to get a full makeup on very quickly can result in mistakes or a sloppy makeup application.

Building an Eye Design

The way to construct an eye design is to place colors across the eye that blend one over the other so that you can't see where one stops and another starts. The basic concept is to shade the eye to accent its shape or change its shape by the progression of light to dark colors across the eye. I will explain step by step how you can use either one eyeshadow or up to five different eyeshadows to create a well-blended, beautiful eye design. Whether you use one, two, three, four, or five different eyeshadows, they become a full design when worn with eyeliner, temple contour, blush, and mascara.

One-color eye design. One *soft* shade of eyeshadow is applied all over the eye area from the lashes to just under the eyebrow. Hopefully you will not wear only a splash of color over the eyelid and ignore the rest of the eye area. This design blends a soft, subtle color all over the eye, leaving no patches of skin showing through. When applying this first color it is easy to find the lid area; it is more difficult to find the underbrow area. Place the color from the lashes to the crease, being sure that you do not extend the color into the teardrop or out beyond the lashes. Also be certain there are no patches of skin showing through at the inside corner of the eye or next to the lashes.

The underbrow area is a little more complicated. This area starts at the instep of the eye (see diagram F), where the eyebrow begins, next to the bridge of the nose. If you had applied a nose contour, that's where the contour color would have stopped and the underbrow shadow placement started. Regardless of whether or not you've contoured the nose, the underbrow color starts here; with the nose right there, it provides a natural indentation that keeps the front edge of your eyeshadow from looking too obvious. Apply the underbrow color from this inner corner by the nose down to the crease, and up into the eyebrow itself, blending out and across to the end of the brow and out into the temple contour. That's why the temple contour is there; so that you won't see where the eye makeup starts and stops at the back of the eye.

I usually encourage using an eyeliner and temple contour when eyeshadows are applied, but for this simple design temple contour is not necessary. Because the eyeshadow for this one-color eye design should be so soft or subtle, there wouldn't be much of a hard edge at the back corner of the eye where the eyeshadow stops. This one color blended over the entire eyelid and underbrow should be a light tan, neutral taupe, beige, pale mauve brown, or pale gray. Whatever the color is, it should definitely not be an obvious color.

Two-color eye design. The lighter color of the two eyeshadows you are using is applied fully on the eyelid and the other color is applied over

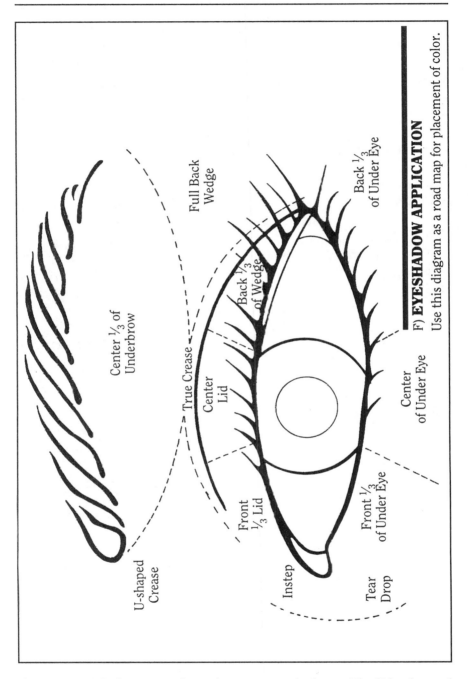

F) EYESHADOW APPLICATION

Use this diagram as a road map for placement of color.

the entire underbrow area from the crease to the brow. The lid color and underbrow color in this design meet at the crease but do not overlap. Generally speaking, the underbrow color is a shade or two darker than the lid color. It is not a distinctly different color, just a different shade. The lid can be a taupe, beige, or tan shade and the underbrow can be a deeper shade of taupe, beige, or tan. It is okay to wear a muted rose or soft shade of pink as long as it doesn't make your eyes look irritated. Bright or shiny shadows can look dated and make the brow bone look more prominent and heavy. A liner completes this design, but once again a temple contour is an option.

Which color goes where? When trying to choose which eyeshadow color goes where, there are two general rules to always keep in mind: the bigger the eyelid area, the darker or deeper the color can be; and the smaller the eyelid area, the brighter or lighter the color can be. If the eyelid area is already prominent or large, it isn't necessary to make it appear any bigger. If the eyelid area is small, it is appropriate to make it larger by wearing a lighter color.

This same general rule applies for the underbrow area. The smaller the area between the crease and the eyebrow, the lighter the color can be in this area. The larger the area between the crease and the eyebrow, the deeper or darker the color can be. If the area under the eyebrow is about the same as that of the lid, the choice is yours; either may look fine.

Caution: *Never use shiny white, bright white, or iridescent colors anywhere on the eye. They are too obvious, glaring, and can make the eye look wrinkled.*

Building a More Dramatic Eye Design

Three-color eye design. Start by applying either the one- or two-color eye design. Once you have done that, add your third color choice in either a back wedge *or* a U-shaped crease design. What, you may well be asking, are the back wedge and U-shaped crease designs? They are the most classic ways I've found to shape and define the eyes. Because the next two designs also use the back wedge and U-shaped crease, I'll describe them after I've suggested color combinations for all of them.

For the three-color eye design, the lid and underbrow colors are softer and less intense than the back wedge or U-shaped crease colors. The crease color can be a deep shade of brown, charcoal, mahogany, sable, or red-brown. To complete this design you need to include a temple contour and eyeliner.

Four-color eye design. Starting again with the one- or two-color eye design, add a U-shaped crease color *and* a back wedge. When both a U-shaped crease color and a back wedge color are used, the back wedge color is more intense or darker than the crease color. The U-shaped crease color can be a deep shade of brown, charcoal, mahogany, sable, or redwood. The back wedge can be a deep burgundy, slate, gray-brown, dark brown, or black. To complete this design, include a temple contour color and an eyeliner.

Five-color eye design. Starting with the one- or two-color eye design, add a back wedge color and a U-shaped crease color. The last step is to apply a true crease color (see diagram F). For this extremely intricate eye design the lid and underbrow are the lightest shades, the U-shaped crease color is darker, and the wedge and true crease color are the darkest shades of all.

How to Apply the Back Wedge and Full Back Wedge

The back wedge is an accent color that shades either the back third corner of the lid only or the back third corner of the lid extending slightly into the underbrow area and temple contour. When only the back third of the lid is shaded it is called a back wedge. When the back third corner of the lid is shaded, and then you blend that color carefully into the crease and up into the back half or third of the underbrow color and contour color, it is called a full back wedge (see diagram G).

The trick to getting the back wedge on correctly is to be in complete control of the color placement. Be sure to knock the excess off your brush and place the color on in very small strokes only over the back third of the lid. The problem with control is keeping the color on the back third of the lid area only. If you don't know how to handle the brush, you can end up accidentally having the back wedge take up more than half of the eyelid or blend out into the temple area, which would then make it a full back wedge, and at least for this design, that is not where you want it.

Start by applying your shadow to the back wedge area only on the back third of the lid. Once that is applied, without putting more powder on the brush, blend the back wedge shadow from the lid out toward the underbrow and temple contour area. It is essential that you not make this full back wedge look like a stripe or a smudge (see diagram H). It is also important that the most intense placement of color is on the back third of the lid and not the underbrow. As you blend the full back wedge into place out on the underbrow, this area should be the softest part of the color placement.

Another hint to doing the full back wedge correctly is to watch the angle of your brush as you blend the color from the lid toward the underbrow area. If you place your color straight up at a 90-degree angle, you will look like you drew on wings. The softer the angle, the softer the appearance, so be certain you blend out and slightly up from the lid area toward the underbrow. The full back wedge color should never reach the brow itself.

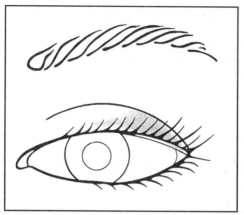

G) **WEDGE**

Shade the back $\frac{1}{3}$ of the lid only.

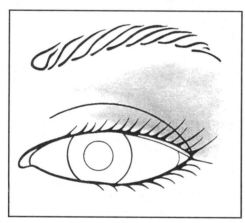

G) **FULL BACK WEDGE**

Shade from back $\frac{1}{3}$ of lid out to the back $\frac{1}{3}$ of the under-eyebrow. Temple contour blends out back edge of eyeshadow.

The U-shaped Crease

The U-shaped crease design is a wonderful look to achieve but not very easy to accomplish. The wonderful part of this design is that it shades, defines, and creates movement by adding a shadow in a curved flowing motion that follows the natural shape of the eye. The difficult part of this design is blending this crease color across the entire length of the eye without making it look obvious. Add to those two problems the fact that the U-shaped crease color is darker than the lid and underbrow color and you've got an interesting task to complete. But it is well worth it. The U-shaped crease color is a basic eye design to use if you are wearing a full makeup or a more dramatic evening makeup.

The U-shaped crease starts from the front third of the underbrow, sloping downward to the center true crease area and then gradually blending back up again to the back third of the underbrow out into the temple contour. Of course, this sweep of color needs to go on without looking like a stripe across the eye. Concentrate your efforts on the area under the front third of the brow where the U-shaped crease color starts and the dip in the center to the crease, and then decide when to start your blending back up again toward the back third of the eyebrow (see diagram I).

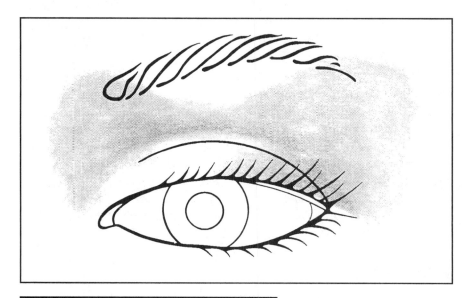

I) U-SHAPED CREASE
This design always includes a Full Back Wedge.

Note: *I have vacillated between calling this design a U-shaped or an S-shaped design. When you look at the finished design it resembles a U, but when applying, it goes on like an S due to the curved shape of the front third underbrow area where the design starts.*

I have a few suggestions for achieving a fail-safe application. The center crease area is always the darkest, so start your brush there and blend out and up to the front third of the underbrow, being careful to keep this area soft and well blended. When you've finished applying the color to the center crease and the front third of the underbrow, place your brush back on the crease and then begin blending up and out to the back third of the underbrow from this center point. The softest part of the design is the front and back third of the underbrow, so be careful not to build up too much color in those areas.

The way to decide when to start blending the back and front part of the U-shaped crease color up from the center of the crease is to first discover where the eyebrow bone starts curving down. Look at your eyes in a mirror. Notice the crease area that curves across your eye (this is also present in Asian women; although the fold is different, the crease area is still there). Notice that the center of the crease area is the highest point and the rest of the crease curves down away from this point in a half-moon shape around the eye. From this high center point, aiming away from where the crease begins curving downward, is where you should begin blending the U-shaped crease color up toward the back third of the underbrow. Or, in the other direction, up toward the front third of the under brow. This gives the illusion of lifting and opening the eye.

Note: *Notice in diagram I that the U-shaped crease color always shades the back third of the lid just as in the back wedge design. This prevents the crease color from looking like a stripe hanging out in mid-air. The difference, then, between the three-color design, which gives you the option of using either a U-shaped crease color or a back wedge color, and a four-color eye design, utilizing* both *the back wedge and the U-shaped crease color, is color selection. When the U-shaped crease color is applied along the back third of the lid, the lid is the same color as the crease. When both the back wedge and U-shaped crease are applied, the back wedge is an entirely different and darker color than that used in the crease.*

True Crease

A five-color eye design adds a true crease color to the full four-color eye design application. This fifth color is a deep color used in the exact fold of the eye that then connects with the back wedge on the lid. The true crease color is placed below the U-shaped crease color along the distinct crease of the eye. The true crease and back wedge are always the most intense color of the eye design. The true crease and the back wedge color are often the same color.

The only trick to applying the true crease color is to make sure there is not a pencil-thin stripe in the crease. It isn't a large area but it shouldn't be too thin either. Follow the crease exactly, starting the brush after the teardrop and taking it all the way through the crease to the back third of the lid where it blends with the back wedge color.

You already know that the lid color should be lighter than the underbrow when the lid is smaller than the underbrow, and that the lid color should be somewhat darker than the underbrow when the lid is larger than the underbrow area. The back wedge and the U-shaped crease should be a darker or richer color than both the lid and underbrow colors. If you use both the back wedge and the U-shaped crease design, the U-shaped crease color should be a softer color than the back wedge. The primary idea is to choose colors that are progressive shades of light to dark in the same color family. Avoid choosing colors that are radically different from each other. That is no small task when you consider that most eyeshadow colors come packaged in groupings that don't work together, such as pink, teal green, and coral, or yellow, purple, blue, and pink.

You will be much better off if you can find neutral shades that work together. A perfect combination would be a beige color on the lid, a slightly darker tan color under the eyebrow, followed by a gray-brown tone in the crease and a slate gray in the back wedge. If you are interested in a slightly more colorful array of shadows, the only *colors* I recommend using are a pale gray-toned lavender on the lid, a pale mauve-taupe shade under the eyebrow, a deep grayish purple in the U-shaped crease, and a dark purple on the back wedge. Always be careful when using eyeshadow colors that aren't neutral. Use only gray or deep colors that do not stand out. If you want to wear a more obvious color, only one obvious color at a time is necessary, and the back wedge is a safe place to apply it.

Remember: *Watch your blending and placement of eyeshadows. Keep in mind that you should be concerned with how each eyeshadow color blends and overlaps into the other instead of where each eyeshadow color starts and stops. What you want is smooth movement so that the eyeshadows are blended over the eye without stripes, lines, streaks, smudges, or smears. To make this whole process as easy as possible, use colors that are easy to blend, and always use the temple contour brush or your sponge to soften the back edge of your eye makeup. To assure yourself guaranteed success, avoid like the plague glittery, iridescent, and shiny eyeshadows. Shiny eyeshadows exaggerate the lines on the eye, making you look wrinkly even when you don't have wrinkles.*

Eye design mistakes to avoid:

1 Do not overcolor the eyes: too many bright colors can be distracting, not attractive.

2 Do not create hard edges: you should not be able to see where one color stops and another starts.

3 Do not wear bright pink or iridescent pink eyeshadows; they make eyes look irritated and tired. Muted pink is an option, but be very, very careful. If it makes the eye look irritated or "red," it isn't the color for you.

4 Do not wear shiny eyeshadows of any kind; they make skin look wrinkled.

5 Do not wear a vivid, bright eyeshadow color all over the eyelid.

6 Do not forget to apply temple contour.

7 Do not wear bright blue, bright green, or bright turquoise eyeshadow.

8 Do not use a bright white or bright color highlighter under the eyebrow bone.

9 Do not forget to knock the excess shadow off your brush before you touch the brush to your eye.

10 Do not forget to use temple contour to help soften the eyeshadows at the back corner of the eye.

Eyeliners

Let's take a short trip down eyeliner memory lane. Between 1960 and 1974 we progressed from wearing heavy liquid liner that swept over the eyelid, ending in wings at the back of the eye, to wearing Twiggy lashes, which were pointy lines drawn vertically from the lower lashes with false eyelashes worn on the lid. Then, somewhere around 1976, the smudge pencils came into fashion. The smudge sticks were great; they were fast and convenient and, sad to say, did just what their name said they would do; they smudged all over the place. Smeared eye makeup was a definite problem.

Then there was the period in the early eighties when a fashionable eye was one where the liner was placed on the inside rim of the eye. We were told that placing the pencil here would make the white of the eye appear whiter. Nothing could have been further from the truth. With constant application of a foreign substance in the eye, the resulting irritation left the eye bloodshot and tearing. Plus this lovely effect of lining the inside rim lasted only about one hour and then the color clumped up at the inside corner of the eye and smeared under the eye. During the mid-eighties, eyeliner became a more specific, though soft, line around the outside of the eyes and the pencils were thinner and more reliable. Unfortunately, thin eye pencils, even if they don't smudge as much as fatter pencils do, can still smear and wear off.

Today there are several styles of liner you can choose, but there are some you should consider avoiding and some that last longer than others. What kind of eyeliner should you use? Because of all the problems I just mentioned with regard to pencils, even though they are easier, I rarely recommend them for eyelining. Also, pencils are hard to sharpen, which makes it difficult to keep a good point intact, making it harder for you to control the thickness of the line. But that is not so with a brush and a powder. Whenever you're lining the eyes, I strongly recommend using a dark-toned eyeshadow color (any eyeshadow color can work) and a tiny brush. The tiny, thin eyeliner brush allows absolute control over the thickness of the line around the eye. Another benefit to using powder and a brush is that you can always use the powder as an eyeshadow by just changing the brush size.

Do you need to wear eyeliner? If you are wearing eyeshadow I almost always recommend wearing eyeliner, unless the lid and eyelashes are covered by the underbrow. Eyeliner is a basic part of an eye design because it is a key factor in shaping the eye and making the eyelashes look thicker. If you are not wearing eyeshadow and only mascara, eyeliner is an option but not necessary. When you are wearing mascara and no eyeshadow, be sure to line the eyes with only a very soft, well-blended eyeshadow color.

How do you apply a powder eyeliner? Choose a dark or intense shade of eyeshadow. Always line the eyes last—after all the other eyeshadows are applied. Use a thin, slightly stiff brush. Whether you use your powder wet or dry (either is fine, but dry is softer and wet is more dramatic), stroke the brush through the color, keeping the bristles together. Do not dab or rub the brush into the color. Move the brush across the shadow in the direction of the bristles, making sure the form of the brush is not destroyed (see diagram C). Knock the excess color from the brush and then apply the color to the eyelid next to the lashes and under the eye near the lower lashes.

When lining the eyelid make the line a solid, even line, starting thin at the front third of the lid, becoming slightly thicker at the back third of the lid. You can line all the way across the eyelid if you like, from the inside corner to the outer edge, or you can stop the line where the lashes stop and start. Along the lower lashes, line only the outer two-thirds of the eye, with a softer color than the liner you used on the lid. Never line all the way across the lower eyelashes. Always leave some space where the lashes end inside near the tear ducts. Wrapping a complete eyeliner circle around the eye tends to create an eyeglass look and strongly changes the definition and softness. It can make the eyeliner the stronger statement rather than the eye itself, and it is also out of date. It is sometimes recommended that women over forty should not line the inner corner of the eyes either on top or bottom. I think that is a fine suggestion.

How thickly can you line the eye? Thicker eyeliner is definitely in. The sixties look was revived and shows up in magazines all the time, and is a part of Madonna's Marilyn look. Should you follow the fashion or do something more classic? As a general rule, for a safe classic look, the thickness and intensity of the eyeliner is determined by the size of the lid: the larger the eyelid area, the thicker and softer the eyeliner should be. The smaller the eyelid area, the thinner and more intense the liner should be. When your lid doesn't show at all, forget lining altogether. Another important tip for a classic soft eyeliner look is to be sure the lower liner is a less intense color than the upper liner and that the two lines meet at the back corner of the eye.

Should you apply a sixties-looking eyeliner? Unless you are in your twenties and going out dancing for the evening, overexaggerated eyeliner with wings beyond the corner of the eyes is not a good idea. You can use a more definite eyeliner look, but keep it soft by using powder or using a pencil and then applying powder over it.

Which eyeliner color should you use? The general rule for applying a classic shade of eyeliner is to choose a brown, gray, or black eyeshadow. Eyeliner is meant to give depth to the lashes and make them appear thicker. If the liner is a bright or true pastel color, the attention will be focused past the lashes to the colored line as opposed to the more subtle flow of color from dark lashes to dark liner. Test it on yourself. Line one eye with a vibrant color, the other eye with a brown or black, and see which one looks like it has thicker lashes. Then, if all my attempts to convince you have failed, and you still prefer to use bright pastel liners, do so.

You may have seen or heard a dozen other ideas as to how to apply eyeliner. Halfway across the lid, or one-third, or one-fourth, and three-fourths of the way under the lower eyelashes or one-third, or one-fourth, and on and on. You are more than welcome to experiment with all these placements, but I would still encourage you to try the classic way first and see how you like it. Because I believe that the major reason to wear eyeliner is to shape the eye and make the eyelashes look thicker and deeper, I feel it is important to line the lashes. You can always line with a very soft color if you are concerned about overdefining the eyes, but I am not convinced that these "adjusted" lengths of placement look very natural.

Eyeliner mistakes to avoid:

1 Do not use greasy pencils to line the eye; they smear and smudge.

2 Do not use brightly colored eyeshadows to line the eye.

3 Do not extend the liner beyond the corner of the eye.

4 Do not make the eyeliner the most obvious part of the eye design.

5 Do not line the rim of the eye; it is out-of-date, messy, and unhealthy for the eye.

6 Do not use brightly colored pencils or eyeshadows to line the eye; they are distracting and unfashionable. All you'll see is the color and not your eye.

7 Do not forget to apply a small amount of eyeshadow over your eyeliner pencil to help set it.

8 Do not apply thick eyeliner to small or close set eyes.

9 Do not use eyeshadow as an eyeliner without the proper brush.

Drippies

Last but not least, after the eye design and eyeliner are completed, check for drippies under the eye and on the cheek. Drippies are those little powder flakes that fly off the brush and land on the cheek. Knocking off the excess from the brush every time helps prevent drippies, but there will always be flakes that end up where they don't belong. The best way to go after drippies is to use your sponge and simply wipe them away. Some makeup artists recommend applying the foundation, highlighter, and eye design and then checking for drippies. If you do this, your next step is to touch up your foundation and apply the blush and contour. Drippies can easily smear a neatly applied makeup so this order of application should definitely be considered.

Mascara

Mascara is a wonderful invention and is considered basic to any kind of makeup application. Many experts, including myself, say that if you're not wearing any other makeup but still want to wear something, wear mascara. On the other hand, many of us—and I'm guilty of this one too— get carried away and wear way too much mascara.

Women overdo lashes because the cosmetics industry tells us loudly and clearly that long lashes are to be coveted. When we think of applying more mascara, visions of longer, thicker lashes immediately come to mind. Depending on what you mean by *more*, you may be applying too much. Too much mascara increases chances that the mascara will flake, chip, or smear and that the lashes will appear hard and spiked. The eyelashes can only take so much weight and the excess weight can break them. Gunked-up lashes with tons of mascara do not resemble long, thick lashes—they resemble gunked-up lashes.

The desire for longer, more noticeable lashes brings up the ever-popular device that curls the lashes by squeezing them into a bent-upward shape. The problem with curling lashes is that it can place the lashes at a severe angle, which looks unnatural, and while it makes lashes look longer, it ends up breaking and pulling them out. Doesn't that defeat the purpose of making your lashes look longer?

Mascara comes in two basic types: waterproof and water-soluble. The problem with water-soluble mascaras is that many of them *don't come off* all that easily with water. Other than those, there are great water-soluble mascaras that do come off easily and build long, thick lashes (refer to *Don't Go to the Cosmetics Counter Without Me* for specific recommendations). Waterproof mascara causes problems because it doesn't dissolve in water. In order to remove this type of mascara you must pull and wipe at the eye, which sags the skin and can pull out lashes. I understand the desire to go swimming and have your makeup protected, but I still think it causes more headaches in the long run. The final decision is up to you.

By the way, due to a lot of scratched corneas, it is hard to find mascaras that contain fibers anymore. Nowadays, most lash-lengthening-type mascaras are not all that different in formulation from any other mascara.

Apply mascara to the lower lashes by holding the wand perpendicular to the eye and parallel to the lashes, which prevents your getting mascara on the cheek. It also makes it easier to reach the lashes at both ends of the eye. Both the traditional application of mascara—round-brushing the upper lashes from the base of the lash up, and holding the wand perpendicular at the edges and for the lower eyelashes—can get all the lashes around the entire eye. Keep an old, cleaned-up mascara wand in your makeup bag to be used for removing mascara clumps and separating lashes.

Have you ever had mascara end up on the eyelid or under the eye while you're applying it? Mascara landing on the skin can often be simply taken care of. Wait until it dries completely and then chip the mascara away with a cotton swab or your sponge. Most of it will just flake off, with very little repair work needed. Always check for mascara smudges; they can look very sloppy and distracting.

Should you extend the longevity of your mascara tube? If you want to, there are a few possibilities that can make a big difference. The tendency for the mascara tube to dry up can be alleviated by not overpumping the wand into the tube in an attempt to build up mascara on the brush. All that pumping action really accomplishes is pumping air into the tube, which makes the mascara dry up faster. Another solution is to avoid the wider-bristled mascara brushes. In order to accommodate the wider brush, the tube opening needs to be larger and this allows more air to get inside, causing the mascara to dry out faster. Don't be fooled by the promise that wider bristles will make lashes longer, because that is not the major thing that affects application. If anything, when the brush applicator is too big it becomes clumsy to use, and then it's harder to get the lashes at the corners without making mistakes.

Many experts say you shouldn't add water to your mascara tube and that is probably a good recommendation. However, I do on occasion stretch the life of my mascara by adding a mere drop of distilled water to the tube. I've increased the life of my mascara for at least a month by doing this, but, once again, the decision is yours. This, of course, applies only to water-soluble mascara.

Mascaras are not supposed to smudge, flake, or clump. It is not your fault if they do. Price does not tell you anything about a mascara's application. Drugstore mascaras can be as good as anyone else's, and sometimes even better.

Blue Eyelashes?

As I'm sure you've already guessed, I'm not going to suggest that you use blue, purple, or green mascara. Aside from the fact that no one has purple or blue lashes naturally, this book deals more with classic makeup looks—and purple eyelashes would hardly create a traditional look.

Mascara is meant to enhance the eyes, not the lashes. Multicolored mascaras, like colored eyeliners, become a distraction and can make you look at the lashes separate from the eye. If you want the lashes to appear thick and shape the eye, it is important that the mascara be of similar intensity and color as the eyeliner so that they flow from one to the other without separation. The only time to wear pastel mascaras is for a more fun, untraditional look. With that information, the only decision left is when to use black, dark brown, or light brown.

Determine the color intensity of your mascara by the other makeup you're wearing and the color of your lashes. If you're applying black liner and dramatic eye makeup, then use black mascara. A soft daytime makeup is perfect for brown liner and dark brown mascara. If you have blond hair, blond lashes, and blond eyebrows, use light brown mascara and a soft brown liner. A blond woman with very dark brows and dark lashes can use black or dark brown mascara, depending on the intensity of the rest of the makeup.

Mascara mistakes to avoid:

1 Do not overapply mascara and make lashes look clumpy or like thick bar windows.

2 Do not apply colored mascara for a daytime professional look.

3 Do not wear mascara that smears; there are those that don't.

4 Do not forget to apply mascara evenly to lower lashes.

5 Do not use waterproof mascaras on a daily basis; they are too difficult to get off.

Eyebrows

No aspect of makeup has gone through such dramatic fashion changes as eyebrow styles. Eyebrows are as representative of each fashion decade as clothes are. We've gone from overtweezed, pencil-thin, tortured brows to overdrawn, thickly penciled brows to, finally, a very soft, full, virtually tweezer-free eyebrow. The idea is to think of eyebrows as being natural in appearance with no obvious tweezed line etched into the shape.

A full natural eyebrow is not only more attractive, it is also easier to keep up. Of course, that doesn't mean you should have one thick line of eyebrow growing across the nose from one hairline to the other. We are talking natural, not Neanderthal. There is a middle ground between Groucho Marx and Greta Garbo when it comes to the shape of your brows.

Discovering the best shape for your eyebrow without sacrificing the thickness is what you want to accomplish. The shape and length of the eye itself is framed by the arch, length, and thickness of the eyebrow. As much as the shape of a moustache can change the appearance of a man's face, so does the shape of an eyebrow affect the appearance of the eyes. For example, if you tweeze too much off the front part of the eyebrow, the eyes will appear smaller. Or if you tweeze too much away from under the eyebrow, increasing the distance between the eye and the eyebrow, you can look as if you are permanently raising your eyebrow in a surprised expression.

Deciding which hairs to leave and which ones to remove makes the difference between an attractively shaped brow and a misshaped one. You can use a pencil and diagram to help you line up the following parameters for shaping your eyebrow. The brow should begin in alignment with the center of the nostril. The arch should fall at the back third of the eye, and although the eyebrow should be as long as possible, it still shouldn't extend into the temple area. The basic rule to follow is that *the front part of the brow should never drop below the back part of the brow.* Allowing this to happen, either with the way you tweeze your eyebrow or the way you draw it on, makes you look like you're frowning or overemphasizes the downward movement of the back part of the eye (see diagram J).

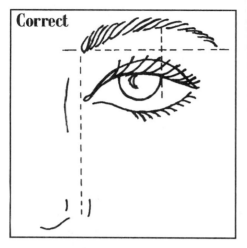

Correct

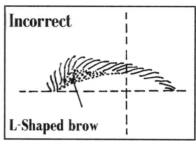

Incorrect

L-Shaped brow

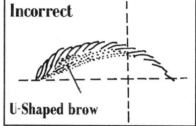

Incorrect

U-Shaped brow

EYEBROW

The eyebrow is correct when the arch falls over the back 1/3 of the eye and the front 1/3 of the brow starts from the center of the nostril.

L-SHAPED BROW

Problem: Arch is over front $\frac{1}{3}$ of brow.
Cure: Grow in or powder indicated area.

U-SHAPED BROW

Problem: No arch.
Cure: Grow in or powder indicated area.

Incorrect

Over-Extended Brow (back)

OVER-EXTENDED BROW (back)

Problem: Back $\frac{1}{3}$ of brow is lower than front $\frac{1}{3}$ of brow.
Cure: Grow in or powder indicated area. Tweeze indicated area.

OVER-EXTENDED BROW (front)

Problem: Front $\frac{1}{3}$ of brow is lower than back $\frac{1}{3}$ of brow.
Cure: Tweeze indicated area.

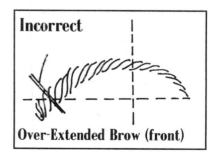

Incorrect

Over-Extended Brow (front)

To apply eyebrow color, use a soft-textured powder (either an eyeshadow or a powder designed for the brow) and a soft wedge brush, following the basic shape of the brow and using the same guidelines as for tweezing. I never recommend using eyebrow pencils. They can produce a greasy look, mat the eyebrow hair, and too often end up looking like a leftover from another decade. If you are presently penciling your eyebrow, seriously consider changing. If it doesn't look absolutely natural, don't do it. Better to go without any eyebrows than to be adorned with a line of pencil above your eye.

To apply the powdered brow color, brush the brow up with an old toothbrush and then apply the color with an angled wedge brush, filling in the shape of the brow in between the hairs where needed. If you need to reshape your eyebrow, a good rule to follow on where to place the color along the brow is, If your eyebrows are set high, away from the eye area, place the color directly under the eyebrow. The closer the brow is to the eye area, the more you should fill in the color toward the top of the brow. As much as possible, only work with the hair that is there. The idea is to shade rather than draw on an eyebrow. Do not place your brow color, whether it is pencil or powder, more than one-quarter inch away from where the natural hair growth stops. It simply looks very fake and accentuates the fact that there is no brow there in the first place. What you want is the suggestion, the shadow of a brow—not a line and not an obvious application of color.

What color eyebrow shadow should you use? Match the eyebrow color to the exact color of the brow rather than to your hair color or a color you think would look better than what already exists. You don't want to see a separation between the eyebrow hair and the shadow used to fill it in. If you have pale eyebrows and want to darken the brow color, use a soft shade of brown that is as close to your brows' natural color as possible. If you have red hair and brown eyebrows, using a red pencil or red-brown powder will look unnatural. A woman with blond eyebrows may use a slightly darker blond or taupe color on her brows to make them visible.

What if you don't have any hair at all where the eyebrow is supposed to be? This is the only time that you would apply a brow color that matches your hair color. Use the wedge brush and powder to follow the bone above the eye, using whatever little hair is there. Usually there's enough shape to create a natural, shaded impression of a brow. Use a light touch, short, quick motions, and avoid the temptation to exaggerate the shape, arch it severely, or extend it into the temple. Downplay the fact that there is no hair and don't overexaggerate it with a strong, eye-catching line. Also, don't place a highlighter or light-colored eyeshadow under the brow to delineate further the placement of the brow color. Something dark next to something light makes it look even more prominent. Use what you have as the basis for any makeup application; do not make any obvious, theatrical changes.

An option for sparse, light-colored eyebrows or eyebrows you want to make look thicker is to use the new colored eyebrow gels that are available at many cosmetics counters. These products look like mascara but they are much less thick and heavy. You apply the color through the brow in much the same fashion as you apply mascara to the eyelashes. There are many colors to choose from, so you want to be sure to get one that matches the eyebrow color. Brush the wand through the brow, being careful not to get it on the forehead or have the brow standing straight up. It will take you a few times to get the hang of it. You might have trouble at first controlling the amount of gel from the tube to the brow. If you want to have your brows look fuller, give this one a try—it really works.

Eyebrow mistakes to avoid:

1 Do not overtweeze or tweeze at all if you don't have to.

2 Do not use eyebrow pencil or eyeliner pencil to fill in your eyebrows unless you are adept at making it look very soft and shaded.

3 Do not apply eyebrow powders that are different from your own eyebrow color, no matter how sparse they are. Always match your existing brow color.

4 Do not overstate the shape of the brow; minimal brow alteration is the best.

5 Do not apply brow color that is noticeable or has a drawn-on look.

6 Do not forget that eyebrow color should look shaded and soft, not like a straight, hard line.

Lipstick and Lip Pencil

Most of you already know this one, but I've also talked to enough women to know that this next comment needs to be made. Simply put, if you're wearing makeup, your lips will need lipstick—not lip *gloss*, but lip*stick*. Lip gloss doesn't last, but lipstick does. Lip gloss is for a sheer temporary look or for teenagers who are not supposed to be wearing makeup. Lipstick (cream lipstick, not iridescent) is for a polished and put-together look that can last at least until your second cup of coffee. Naked lips with made-up eyes or cheeks can look like when applying your makeup you forgot you had a mouth. For the sake of balance, remember your mouth.

When you wear lipstick, a lip brush or lip pencil is an optional mouth accessory. Lip pencil helps to draw a definitive edge around the mouth to follow when applying lipstick, and a lip brush helps control your application. The lipstick tube itself is too big for some lips and too small for others. If your lips are small it is best to use a lip brush; if your lips are large the only reason to use a lip brush is for improved accuracy.

When using a lip pencil, always place the color on the actual outline of your mouth. Do not use corrective techniques that make the mouth look larger or longer, especially for daytime makeup. If you try to change the outline of your mouth with a lip pencil by drawing it on the outside of the lips, two hours later, when your lipstick wears off, the lip liner, which lasts longer than the lipstick, will still be in place and it will look like you missed your lips. Always line the lips following the actual shape, then fill in with your lipstick color, using either the tube or lipbrush.

Lip pencils stopped being an obvious dark, brown, or definite line around the mouth over a decade ago. (Brown lip pencils and lipsticks weren't attractive colors when they were in fashion.) They made a brief comeback a year or two ago, but the fashion magazines have regained their senses. Your lip pencil should not make an obvious line that shows up as a colored border around the lipstick. The goal is to have the lipstick and lip pencil meld so that you can't see where one starts and the other stops.

To help your lipstick last longer, apply the lip pencil all over the lip area, including the outline of the lips, and then apply your lipstick color over it. The benefit of doing this is to place a more permanent color on the lips, so the lipstick won't wear off as fast as it normally does. As you already know, there is no such thing as all-day lipsticks.

When choosing the color of lipstick to wear, follow these basic rules. Thinner lips need to wear brighter, more vivid colors and avoid darker shades. Deeper colors on thin lips makes the mouth look severe and harsh. Larger lips can wear just about any color, but the softer, brighter shades are more fashionable and usually more versatile than darker or vivid colors, which can make your lips too prominent. Brighter colors may take a bit of getting used to, but they truly make the mouth look softer and more attractive.

How can you stop your lipstick from traveling into the lines around your mouth? The first thing is to stop wearing greasy lipsticks and lip glosses. The greasier the lipstick or lip pencil is, the faster the color will slip into the lines around your mouth. The drier-feeling lipsticks are best for conquering this problem. Powdering the mouth with loose powder before applying the lipstick also helps, but can be a bit messy.

A few years ago some cosmetics companies came out with new products that were supposed to prevent lipstick from bleeding. I tried a lot of these and many never worked. I finally found three that have changed the way I wear lipstick, because now I don't have to worry about my lipstick bleeding: Chanel's Protective Colour Control, Revlon's Color-Lock, and Coty's Stop-It. Of course, Chanel's is the most expensive, but it's not necessarily the best; they all work equally well.

There is no truth to the story you may have heard that using a lipstick brush helps keep the lipstick on longer. Why the brush would serve this purpose has never been explained to me in a manner that makes any logical sense. Lipstick stays on longer when you put on a lot of lipstick, wear strong vivid colors that are not greasy, and avoid wearing lip glosses.

Is there a difference between lipsticks? Yes, there are vast differences between lipsticks. As you probably already know from experience, lipstick colors and textures can vary within the same cosmetics line. Some are creamy, others are dry, greasy, shiny, flat, melt easily, go on sticky, smeary, evenly, thick, thin, and combinations thereof. The lipsticks I recommend go on creamy, in an even layer that doesn't smear or look thick. The only way to discover this for yourself is to be patient and try on the colors you like and see how they feel. But whatever you do, avoid wearing shiny lipsticks, particularly if you are an adult. Shiny lipsticks can make lips look dry and cracked. It is also a much more attractive look to have your lips shine from a creamy smooth lipstick than from iridescence.

Note: *If your lipstick has a tendency to cake or get dry as the day goes by, you will want to avoid reapplying your lipstick over semi-worn-off lipstick. Wipe off all your lipstick first and then reapply your lipstick. You may also want to apply a bit of gloss under your lipstick if the problem of caking persists.*

Lipstick and lip pencil mistakes to avoid

1 Do not use a pencil that is a contrasting color to your lipstick; it is out-of-date and can look severe.

2 Do not exaggerate or change the shape of your mouth with lip pencil or your lipstick; it will inevitably look like you missed your mouth with the lipstick.

3 Do not use lip gloss in place of lipstick during the day; it can bleed and won't last as long as lipstick can.

4 Do not apply a lipstick that is a different color tone from the rest of your makeup colors. For example, if you are wearing blue-tone blush and eyeshadows, wear a blue-tone lipstick.

5 Do not wear iridescent lipstick; when it wears off it can look dry, white, and caked.

Custom Blending

If a foundation is blended for you and you only, will that get you the best shade? What about custom-blended eyeshadows, powders, blushes, and lipsticks? Many cosmetics companies nowadays offer all of these products supposedly designed just for you. This new style of selling makeup is very enticing. The customer service interaction is impressive. All sorts of products are supposedly mixed and matched just for your skin color and needs. The notion is that there are only so many ready-made shades and you might be better off having one custom blended. Unfortunately, it sounds like a better idea than it is. The major problem with custom-blended cosmetics is you are left to the expertise of the salesperson and we all know how reliable that can be. I bought many so-called perfectly blended custom foundations, lipsticks, and eyeshadows while researching *Don't Go to the Cosmetics Counter Without Me*. Particularly with the foundations, almost 80 percent of them turned out to be the wrong color. There was also a problem with the foundation or other makeup colors the factory eventually made for me. It was not unusual for the color I got back to be different from the one that was blended. (With all due respect, the companies I reviewed were always willing to try again and match the color at their own expense or return my money.)

The other issue is that *custom-blended* does not mean the product is any better. The eyeshadows may still be shiny, the lipsticks greasy, and the blush too dark or too light a shade. With all the shades of makeup products available, in many excellent colors, all this custom work turns out to be more an expensive selling gimmick than anything else. *Custom-blended* items can be just as problematic and time-consuming to shop for as any other type of foundation, blush, eyeshadow, powder, or lipstick.

When should you look for a custom-blended product, particularly foundation and powder? When you have tried many standard foundations and are still frustrated with the color of your foundation. Custom blending is costly and best used as a last resort when nothing else has worked.

Choosing Colors That Work Together

It is obvious from the sheer number of makeup colors available that there is no one universally accepted opinion as to the best way to combine colors. There are so many differing opinions and preferences that it's not only unlikely you will ever find the perfect combination, but unnecessary. Just as there isn't one color combination of clothing you wear everyday, the same is true for your makeup. Yet there are ways to go about making two or three good choices that should solve most of your makeup wardrobe needs. Here are some of the most efficient and aesthetically reliable rules.

Color-dress your face the same way you would color-dress your body. If you wouldn't consider wearing a pink skirt with a blue blouse and an orange jacket, don't wear those colors on your face. This means you should avoid wearing orange lipstick, blue eyeshadow, and pink blush. It even sounds distracting. As much as possible, work monochromatically when using colors for the lips, cheeks, and eyes. Dress your face so it doesn't clash with itself. If your blush and eyeshadows are mauve, taupe-lavender, and gray (blue undertones), the lip color should be in the same blue undertone family. The lipstick, then, can be either pink or mauve or some other soft shade of a blue-undertoned color. If your blush and eyeshadow are rust and peach in color (yellow undertones), the lipstick should be peach, rust, coral, pale orange, or red with yellow undertones.

Dress your face so it doesn't clash with what you wear. Matching makeup to your clothing is important. The same way you wouldn't wear a pair of orange shoes with your pink skirt, do not wear an orange shade of lipstick with your pink outfit. That doesn't mean that if you're wearing a blue skirt you should wear blue eyeshadow any more than it means you should wear blue lipstick. This notion is very outdated and unflattering. Besides, the theory falls apart when you wear a black, navy, or red-and-white-striped outfit. What color eyeshadows are you supposed to wear then—black and red? But the clothes you are wearing will always have a particular color undertone and your makeup colors should coordinate with that tone as much as possible.

The undertone of a color refers to how blue or yellow it is. All colors can have either blue or yellow undertones. For example, when gray has yellow undertones it can appear drab or ashen green; when it has blue undertones it can appear charcoal or slate gray. When brown has blue undertones it may appear rosy brown, mauve-brown, or charcoal-brown; when it has yellow undertones it can appear neutral beige to golden tan or copper. When red has blue undertones it can appear pink, scarlet, or fuchsia; when it has yellow undertones it may appear orange, coral, or peach.

If your wardrobe is mostly neutral, without being overwhelmingly blue or yellow undertoned, you have a lot less to worry about when choosing makeup colors to coordinate with your clothing. Your makeup will blatantly clash with your clothing if it is an obvious color mismatch, as with a pink blouse and an orange lipstick or a peach blouse and a rose blush. Even though grays, blacks, tans, and neutral colors of clothing do indeed have blue and yellow undertones, because they tend to be less obvious they rarely clash with most colors of makeup. It is important to think of makeup as a fashion accessory and follow this rule of matching the undertone of your makeup with the undertone of the clothes you're wearing.

Do not wear makeup (or clothing) colors that are more intense or less intense than you are. For those of you who haven't been "seasoned" yet (discovered what clothing colors are best suited to your skin and hair color), or even if you have been, consider this simple, basic color compatibility idea: if you are blond with fair skin, intense colors like black, cobalt blue, fuchsia, or neon red will overwhelm you. Softer colors like gray, azure blue, or pink will look more balanced. If you have dark hair and dark skin, pale blue or pink will make you look pale and blah. The stronger, more intense blue-tone colors look best on women with dark hair and sallow or black skin.

If you are blond and have dark skin or have dark brown hair with fair skin, stronger blue undertones will be great, but you still do *not* want to go *too* intense. Auburn-haired women with fair skin almost always look better in vibrant, rich colors that are yellow based. Red-haired women with fair skin will want to look for colors that are yellow based and rich tones such as gold, vivid coral, khaki, and brown. Gray-haired women with sallow skin can wear the bright vivid blue-toned colors, and gray-haired women with fair skin can wear softer pastel blue-toned colors. (Yellow tones are not the best for women with gray hair unless they are vivid peach-pink color.)

Choosing color can have its agonies even when you know all the color intensity rules. You need to be cautious not only with how you coordinate your makeup with your clothing, but with how different makeup colors look in combination on your skin. Skin tone has a direct effect on the makeup colors you wear, and the opposite of that is also true: makeup colors have a direct effect on your skin tone. If you are looking for a pink (blue undertone) blush to wear, it is important to realize how that color will make your skin look.

For skin that has strong yellow, brown, or ashen green tones, always avoid reinforcing those skin colors by using those colors on the face. Eyeshadows, lipsticks, or blushes in shades of orange, peach, yellow, chocolate brown, gray-green, rust, khaki, or the like will only make sallow skin appear more sallow and pale. If your skin is ruddy and red in appearance, wearing colors such as pink, purple, blue, red, rose, mauve, and the like will only make the face look more red and more irritated.

Sallow skin is better off wearing blue-undertoned colors. If you have dark hair and sallow skin you are better off with vivid blue-toned colors.

If you have sallow skin with blond or light brown hair, blue-toned pastel colors are best. Ruddy skin tone and blond hair is better off wearing yellow-undertoned pastel colors. Ruddy skin tone and dark brown hair is a good candidate for blue-toned pastels.

For further reference about how to find your best colors read, *Color Me Beautiful* by Carole Jackson or any of Emily Cho's books on fashion. I don't always agree with their makeup or skin care information, but what they know about color and clothes is priceless.

What If My Clothes Are the Wrong Color?

Even if the outfit you want to wear is a color that is not the most flattering for you, it is still necessary to find makeup colors that will not clash. For example, if you wear a vibrant purple outfit and the best colors for you are soft pastels, choose eyeshadows in varying shades of mauve, soft gray, and charcoal with a soft pink blush and lipstick. Those makeup colors will work with your outfit and be soft enough to go with your skin tone.

The same is true for a woman who is wearing earthy, yellow-undertoned colors but should be wearing more vibrant blue-undertoned colors such as hot pink or royal blue. In this situation choose colors of blush and lipstick that are more vivid shades of coral pink with eyeshadows that are a soft tan on the lid and underbrow with a charcoal-gray crease and eyeliner color. Those colors should work with both the outfit and skin tone without clashing.

Is Fashion Awareness for Everyone?

At this point, or even sooner, many of you are probably saying, "I don't want things that are fashionable, I just want to look good." Sorry, it's hard, if not impossible, to have one without the other. For example, you might have looked really good in go-go boots and Nehru jackets twenty-odd years ago, but today chances are they will look out of place. What is fashionable today is directly related to what looks good. Yet within any fashion statement there are lots of clothing options to choose from that will look great on you, and the same follows for makeup. Remember false eyelashes, thick plastic eyeliner, white underbrow highlighter, dark brown color in the crease, and dark brown lipstick? Those are all out of style too. Yet there are dozens of other options that have taken their place that look wonderful today. The goal for you is to find what is comfortable, looks good, and is fashionable all at the same time.

Blue Eyeshadow Should Absolutely Be Illegal

This is the perfect time to mention why blue eyeshadow should absolutely, without question, be illegal. Blue is probably the most misused makeup color women wear, although shiny lime green and bright, shiny pink eyeshadows run a close second, with rosy, orange foundations close behind. Solid blue splashed across the lid, or worse, painted all over the eye from the lashes to the brow, flashes out from the eye area like a neon sign. Blue is a difficult color to blend with any other color, so it always tends to stand out and be more obvious then anything else you may have on. You can see a blue stripe across the lid from across the room! Not the eyes, not the face—just the blue eyeshadow.

In all fairness, I'm referring to a complete solid covering of bright blue eyeshadow over the the eyelid or a bright blue eyeliner, thickly wrapped around the lashes. For some eye designs, a little shading at the back of the eye or an eyeliner of navy or slate gray-blue, if done properly and with restraint, isn't the worse thing I can think of. (See, I really can be flexible.)

If you get compliments on your blue eyeshadow or liner, then you definitely should reconsider how you wear your eye makeup. You want people to compliment *you*, not your eyeshadow. You may also want to take the time to flip through a fashion magazine and notice that none of the fashion layouts (the ads for the fashion designers, not the makeup ads) have models wearing blue eyeshadow, so why are you?

You may have heard someone recently say to you, "Blue eyeshadow is coming back in fashion." First of all, I will believe that when I see Nehru jackets and beehive hairdos making a comeback. And second, although fashion is important, in some cases *fashion* is best ignored. Madonna made wearing bras on the outside of clothes fashionable, and I bet that was a fashion statement you wisely ignored.

A Quick Review

Highlighter: Apply the white highlighter along the inside corner of the eye with your finger or a cotton swab, blending it together with the foundation. If you are using a more flesh-tone highlighter, apply it after the foundation has been blended into place.

Foundation: Apply the foundation in dots over the central area of the face with either your fingertips or sponge. Blend the foundation in place with the sponge. Use the edge of the sponge that doesn't have foundation on it to buff and remove the excess. Foundation blends over the white under the eye and on the eyelid. Avoid placing foundation on or near the jawline.

Brush usage: Knock the excess powder off the brush before applying color to the face and use short, quick blending motions. Never wipe or rub the brush across the face.

Contouring: Do before you apply the blush. Use a medium-size blush brush. Be sure never to place the contour color near the jawline or on the cheekbone.

Blushing: Avoid placing the blush near the eye area. Use a large powder brush and apply the color in downward strokes, moving back toward the ear.

Eyeshadow: The lid color is usually the lightest shade of color and goes on first. Next is the underbrow color, which can be slightly darker, lighter or the same color as the lid color depending on the shape and size of the eye. After those two colors are applied, you can apply either or both the U-shaped crease and back wedge color. These two shadows are the darkest part of the eye design.

Eyeliner: The eyeliner can be the same color as the back wedge or U-shaped crease color. The eyeliner goes on after the entire eye design has been applied. The lower liner blends on softer than the eyelid liner.

Mascara: Use brown, dark brown, or black mascara, and do not overdo.

Eyebrows: Generally it is best not to add eyebrow color if you don't have to, but if the eyebrow is too thin or has been overtweezed, softly and subtly fill it in after the rest of the makeup is in place.

Lipstick and lip liner: If you want, outline your lips first with the pencil and then apply a lipstick that matches the lip liner.

Blending: Check your blending with the sponge and, if possible, check it in daylight. No hard lines or drippies should be visible whatsoever.

Potential Problems

Highlighter problems are caused when you use too little or too much of it under the eye. Too little doesn't give enough coverage and too much makes white rings around the eyes or slips into the lines, looking thick and smeary. Too much moisturizer around the eye or a highlighter that is too greasy can easily slip into the lines around the eyes.

Foundation can be a problem if you apply too much or too little—too little and the rest of the makeup will go on choppy; too much and it will look like a mask. Be careful to blend evenly and do not forget to cover the eyelid, especially the outer third (back corner) next to the eyelashes, the corners of the nose, and around the mouth. To assure the sheerest application, use a slightly damp sponge to apply your foundation. Although I only recommend using a moisturizer under foundation when the skin is dry, you can use a moisturizer to help blend your foundation on even sheerer.

Foundation filling the lines on the face is primarily caused by using too much foundation or too heavy a foundation and then not blending it on thinly enough. Use a lightweight water-based foundation and blend well, using a clean edge of your sponge to go over the lines and pick up any excess foundation. Once the foundation is blended you can apply a light amount of loose powder over the lines to prevent the makeup from slipping into them. Be careful not to use too much powder or your makeup will look caked and thick.

If the face is much lighter or darker than the neck, you will need to choose a color that does not cause a line of demarcation between the neck and the face. In this instance, you need to take into consideration the color of the neck when choosing your foundation color.

Red-brown (blue-toned) colors should not be used for contouring on light or fair skin tones. Red shading can make fair skin look burnt and unnatural. Use tan, taupe, or yellow-brown tones only when contouring. Red-brown shades are a good possibility for women of color.

If you have pale skin, be sure to blend your blush and contour colors well to avoid stripes. You can also increase the area of the temple contour and blush to give the face a bit more color. Just be subtle about it—don't overdo. If you have fair skin, use softer colors of shadows, blush, and lipstick.

Darker shades of skin should use stronger makeup tones. During the summer, if you tan, even though you shouldn't, your colors of makeup will need to be different from the ones you wear during the nontanning months.

When your blush goes on choppy, it's usually due to one of three things: not enough foundation, poor blending technique with the brush from either overblending (which wipes off the foundation) or not knocking the excess off the brush (which puts too much color on the face), or using a blush shade that is too strong or too grainy (which tends to go on heavy and uneven).

If you are wearing the U-shaped crease color, be careful not to use too dark or grainy an eyeshadow color or it will be difficult to blend on softly.

Bright or iridescent pink eyeshadows on the lid will make you look like you've been crying. Shiny eyeshadows will make the eye look more wrinkled than it is. And don't forget to check for drippies after the eye design is complete.

What to Do If You Wear Glasses

Glasses can pose problems only if you don't realize how they can affect makeup. Depending on the type of prescription you wear, the lens will change the appearance of the eye. When the lens magnifies the eye, making the eye look larger, you will need to adapt your makeup so it doesn't appear harsh or overdone. Choose eye colors that are soft, being sure to avoid high-contrasting colors. Also apply the eyeliner more softly in a smudged, less-defined line, and avoid applying a heavy, thick coating of mascara.

If the lens demagnifies the eye, you can increase the color and definition around the eye. But be careful—more color does not mean using blues or greens or leaving hard edges. Shades of blue and green or hard edges with this type of prescription will only look like a small hard edge and a small flash of color.

The frame of your glasses will also affect how you apply makeup. Be sure your blush is placed below the edge of the frame. You don't want the frame to break up the movement or angle of the blush.

How To Shop For Makeup

Shopping for makeup can be very tricky. I am totally sympathetic to this dilemma because I know how messy, time-consuming, and frustrating this can be. There is truly only one way to prevent buying the wrong color. *Try it before you buy it*, and do not buy anything because you were intimidated by the salesperson or because you impulsively decided you need it.

Trying makeup on to test the color only works if you put it on your face without other makeup color. It does no good to put makeup on over your other makeup; all that tells you is how a blush will look when worn over your present blush. Also, do not try makeup on over any other part of your anatomy besides your face. Your arm, wrist, or ear is not your face. Consider it this way—you wouldn't shop for a new item of clothing by putting it on over the clothing you're already wearing, would you? And you wouldn't try a blouse on over your left leg to see if it fits! The same is true for your face. You must experiment with different makeup types and colors on a clean face or a face with only your foundation on to really see the effect of the cosmetics you want to buy.

Judging the Texture of a Powder

One way to judge how a color will go on the skin is by feeling the texture of the powder itself. The drier or softer the feel of the powder, the less intense the application is likely to be. The heavier, greasier, or grainier the feel of the powder, the more thick and intense the application will be. With softer-textured shadows and blush, more color will need to be added to build definition. With heavier-feeling powders, less color is needed to build definition. The greasy, heavy, and grainy-textured powders can be very difficult to blend. Generally speaking, it is best to use these as eyeliners or back wedge colors and nothing else. As a general rule, the heavier a color goes on or feels, the better it will be for eyelining; the softer the color goes on, the better it will be for shading, contouring, and blushing.

Try mixing different textures of blushes and eyeshadows with each other or with a transluscent powder to create new color options. You'll double the colors you have to work with by making them softer or darker.

What's in a Name?

When you buy a cosmetic, you can be confident that a lipstick will be a lipstick and a foundation will be a foundation. However, when you try to buy a color of blush or foundation according to name alone, reality exits and fantasy enters. The color name of a product reflects image, not color. When you spend $10 or $20 on a blush or a contour, Brown doesn't sound as expensive or as exciting as St. Tropez Tan or Terracotta. Foundations may be called Porcelain, but what color is porcelain? My porcelain sink at home is white (well, usually white). Calling a lipstick Cherries Jubilee or Bordeaux is not helping you understand what color shade that is supposed to represent. Choosing color by name is truly frustrating and relatively useless. Choose color according to appearance; how it looks once it's on the face is the only way to make a final decision, which is one of the major reasons I don't recommend mail-order or television-ordered makeup. If at all possible, try it on before you buy it or at least be able to view the color.

Put My Blush Where?

Some women are still skeptical about using an eyeshadow or blush on areas of the face for which the label says it was not intended. What should concern you is whether the eyeshadow is a good color to use as an eyeliner or whether the blush is a good color to apply under the eyebrow. Retailers would love for you to think that there is a vast difference between blushes and eyeshadows and that you can't use a product except for where the label tells you to. Most powders, whether they're called blush or eyeshadow, contain the same ingredients. Anything that would be harmful to your eyes would be specifically indicated on the package. Worry about color choice, not product type or name.

Makeup Bags

Most cloth makeup bags that are used to hold cosmetics are inefficient. Not only is it impossible to find anything in them, many of them can't hold everything—especially when you consider the size of the typical compacts you buy. My suggestion is to purchase a large makeup bag that is clear plastic (so you can easily see what's inside), has enough room to hold all your makeup, and can easily be cleaned. Buy a separate, smaller makeup bag that is also clear plastic to carry a few touch-up items with you in your purse or briefcase. While you're at it, you can start making your makeup bag lighter by throwing out or giving away makeup you don't or won't use but hold on to anyway in case you might.

Where Do You Put on Your Makeup?

Bathrooms can be the worst place to put on your makeup. If they're not steamy and damp, then they are poorly lit. Either invest in good lighting or change locations to the best lighting source in the house. If the kitchen table has the best available light and you're concerned about making a mess or leaving your cosmetics lying around, buy a tray large enough that can transport and store all your makeup.

Choosing a Makeup Artist

I highly recommend taking the time to get your makeup done by a professional makeup artist—and not just once, but several times. Being born female doesn't mean you instinctively know how to put on blush and eyeshadow. It also isn't information handed down from generation to generation. If anything, our mothers had less information than we do. Although getting your makeup done professionally is very important and incredibly helpful, the quality of the work you receive can vary greatly. Be prepared to work with your makeup artist as you would your hairdresser. Remember the haircuts you received when you sat down and told the hairdresser to do whatever he/she felt like?

The following checklist will help you select a trained and qualified makeup artist.

1 *Referrals.* How did Dolores turn out when she went? Check with people you know who have seen the makeup artist you're considering. That way you can have a sense of how they work. If possible, don't rely on newspaper ads or the Yellow Pages.

2 *How does the makeup artist wear her own makeup?* If the artist is a woman, that is, her own makeup application can reflect the style, technique, and flare she uses for applying makeup in general. Is her makeup something you'd wish to emulate or something you pray she doesn't do to you? That isn't necessarily a definitive sign, but remember, we're looking for a process to narrow down the choices with. If the makeup artist is a man, ask to see examples of his work.

3 *When starting, does the artist ask you about your lifestyle?* Do you work in an office? Stay home with the children? Have any known allergies to makeup? Another really good set of questions to be asked is, How would you like to see yourself? and How much makeup do you feel comfortable wearing? If the artist seems genuinely concerned about you as opposed to the products she needs to sell to you, then you just may be in good hands. You want your makeup done, not a sales presentation.

4 *Check the artist's background as to where she studied or who she trained under.* Experience isn't everything, but it's good information to have when making a decision between one professional and another. Do you really want someone doing your makeup who was selling shoes a few weeks ago?

In the long run, the worst that can happen when you see a makeup artist is that you won't like the work, and then you can always wash it off. But the chances are that even if you don't like everything, you will at least learn something from the experience. Learning what you don't like as well as learning what you do like is all a part of a complete makeup education.

Note*: If you get your makeup done for free at the cosmetics counters I recommend that you tip the salesperson (about $3 to $5 is appropriate) if you don't buy anything. Separate from my feelings about the misleading information and overexaggerated claims the salespeople are trained to say when they are applying your makeup, they are performing a valuable service. I would never encourage anyone to buy cosmetics for the sake of the cosmetics salesperson's commission, which isn't much anyway, but a tip in recognition for the service, when we aren't buying* *anything, is polite. After all, we tip cab drivers and waiters for doing less than the service we sometimes get from someone who has taken the time to do our makeup. I'm not referring to the times when a salesperson is helping you find a lipstick, foundation, or skin care routine, but rather a complete skin care and makeup application, and only when the service is courteous.*

What To Discuss With Your Makeup Artist

1 *How do you normally wear your makeup?* Once you explain how much makeup you're used to wearing, the artist can get a good idea of how much makeup you will feel comfortable putting on. For example, if you are not used to wearing a foundation, then perhaps wearing only a mini-application of foundation will be best. If you are used to wearing only one eyeshadow, then perhaps it is best to move on to the two-color eye design before trying the back wedge or U-shaped crease color or whatever design series they use.

2 *What is a typical or major color in your (seasonal) wardrobe?* This will help you decide which color direction to focus on. Quite frequently you will have both colors in your wardrobe, blue and yellow undertones, which may mean both makeup color families are necessary for you. If you are a beginner with makeup, start by choosing the color tones that are dominant in your closet.

3 *How do you want to look? Or, what do you need this makeup for?* This will give your artist an idea of how intensely or conservatively you will want to wear your makeup. A more dramatic effect requires more color and defining; a casual, natural-looking makeup requires less. What do you need this makeup for? Work? Social event? If the makeup is for daytime business you will want to wear a more natural look. If it's for an evening out and your clothes are more dramatic, then the makeup should be more dramatic.

4 *Make sure it is okay with the artist that you can ask questions.* As your makeup is being applied you want to get full explanations on what each item is for and how crucial it is for the overall makeup look. If after each item you're told that you can't do your makeup without this essential step, do not buy a thing, you are getting a snow job, not a makeup lesson. If you are spending most of your time discussing products and not makeup-application techniques, you will want to find yourself another makeup artist.

How to Deal with Cosmetics Salespeople

Keep these few things in mind next time you're perusing the cosmetics counters.

The cosmetics salesperson is not necessarily an authority. She is trained to sell a product or, more accurately, she is trained to sell a lot of products. Be conscious that much of what you will be told are sales pitches and not factual information. Also understand that none of that is the salesperson's fault; it is simply the way she earns her living.

No matter what you're being told, if for one moment you think you won't do it, don't buy it. You can reconsider and buy it the next time you're in the store. I promise you the chances are they won't run out.

There is no such thing as "This product won't work without that product"; it sounds convincing, but it is never true.

The more fabulous or elaborately scientific the claim or name of a particular product sounds, regardless of price, the more certain you can be that you will be wasting your money.

Do not approach or allow yourself to interact with a salesperson you feel intimidated by. That is true no matter what you are buying in life. If you don't feel comfortable you will make mistakes, either by buying too much or walking away and not buying what you need.

There is no truth to the superiority of one line over another. The superiority of a cosmetic is not in the brand name but in how the individual product works for you. One counter is the same as the next until you try the stuff on your face and see how it looks and feels and compares to the others.

They're Out to Get Our Children

I think this all started with the Barbie doll. That chesty little clothing monger whose outfits and makeup are eternally perfect. Her hair and makeup is always neatly in place no matter what we do to it. Barbie's been handed down from sister to sister to sister before showing any sign of wear and tear. Even when Ken came along, no matter what nasty things we made them do, her makeup never smeared and her hair was still in place.

The message starts when we are very young that there is some mysterious beauty perfection attainable with a little added something that is not ours naturally. Television advertises it and our mothers unwittingly reinforce it. Our own moms make subtle comments about how we would look better with a little more of this thing or a lot more of the other thing. The idea that we looked fine just the way we were was rarely voiced. Maybe they were afraid we would grow up and go to work with scraped knees or dirty cheeks, or maybe they were only projecting their own insecurities. How many of us have a clear picture of watching our own mothers spend endless hours tending to their hair, adjusting their lipstick, fastidiously applying their eye makeup, and then exhaustedly wiping it off with cold cream or rinsing it off with soap or a cleanser at the end of the day. My mother's dark greasy eyes are as vivid an image to me as her perfectly made-up face.

On the other hand, there were those of us who had moms who never wore makeup, who believed lipstick and blush were the devil's handmaidens. It happened sometime after we started getting our periods. Out of nowhere we had the urge to play with makeup. We were probably testing our femininity and sexuality to see what it felt like being a woman. Once we began experimenting with makeup the problems followed. Often we were punished for the thought of wanting to wear makeup even more than for the actual red lips or blued lids we were caught with. Cosmetics made us look like sluts and that was intolerable. Wouldn't you know it—damned if we did and damned if we didn't.

There are also those mothers who give their children no structure or information around their appearance or sexuality. Young girls wearing heavy, overdone makeup can be seen everywhere. Young girls bombarded with the intensity of MTV and peer pressure are taught, from this unloving source, what it takes to be attractive and special. The necessity for guidance from a loving, supportive parent who recognizes how vulnerable a child's self-esteem and need for self-acceptance can be, is not only crucial, but fundamental.

As confusing as the messages were from our parents, the constant theme of not being okay the way we are is a media standard for both ourselves and our children. The pulsating pictures on TV and in magazines and newspapers send us repeated images of happy, sexually satisfied, perfect-looking people. These are powerful influences reminding us of what we need to do or have in order to be complete. Making us need something more or other than what we have is the most successful marketing tool of all.

This problem of being happy with ourselves just the way we are isn't only for us adults, who have our own insecurities and lack of self-esteem to over come. The issue is, do we want our children bombarded with the same disregard for inner human values and overemphasis on the artificially created exterior?

Children start very young to dress up in the images conveyed by the media and often we are helpless to stop them. Perhaps we, as parents and teachers or friends, forgot to praise the young people in our lives for being lovable no matter what they did or how they did it. Whether a child spills milk or gets straight A's, they need to be reassured that what is precious about each of us is separate from what we do. Though even if we had told our children, they might not have heard. The noise of our own lack of self-worth and the TV blasting in the background probably prevented the communication from getting through.

Perhaps the answer is awareness and an inner voice that is louder and stronger than what we are used to hearing. And if Brooke Shields is happy, it isn't because of her face, hair, or figure, it's because her mother loved and praised her for being alive and nothing else. Being beautiful doesn't make anyone happy. We all know plenty of unhappy *beautiful* people. If we remind ourselves and the smaller ones around us of how wonderful we all are just the way we are, then the world would be a much safer place for our egos to live in. I vote for strong self-images, love of the natural inner and outer selves that starts when we are very young and lasts forever.

Does Makeup Make Us Sexy?

The ever-popular question—do women wear makeup for men or other women—has become obsolete. Women wear makeup for many reasons; a professional look at work, socially when going out with other women, to support their own egos, to enhance their self-esteem, *and* for the purposes of attracting the opposite sex. The more provocative question is, does wearing makeup make us more alluring to men? Are we sexier with or without makeup? The answer is yes and no!

Just applying makeup, even a well-applied makeup, doesn't automatically translate to a visage that would be defined as either sexy, intriguing, provocative, glamorous, or any of those words we associate with an enticing sexual appearance. Although looking sexy is extremely difficult to describe in words, given the wide variety of opinions on the subject of what is sexy, we all know it when we see it. And we see it all the time, almost every day of our lives from the time we are small until we are old. We see it exemplified by almost every actress, model, and female spokesperson on television, movies, covers of record albums, magazines, and advertisements. These very visible women, portraying every imaginable role from lawyers to villains, and representing every imaginable product from cars to soft drinks, in various stages of dress and undress, are all artistically blushed, shaded, contoured, and lipsticked, and extremely sexy. No matter how natural we (or men) may think they look, they aren't, at least not when it comes to their faces. Makeup without question, to one degree or another, can be part of a sexy appearance, but outside of the media it doesn't always look as alluring as we had hoped.

Can you be sexy without makeup? Of course. Can you be more sexy with makeup? Maybe. It depends on the situation and what image you are trying to create. The problem is that the women who want to create this type of enticing, come-hither look for themselves often don't succeed. Many women erroneously believe that looking sexy means layering more makeup on and that's a problem. Gunked-up mascara, heavily lined eyes, stripes of blush, and thick foundation are not sexy.

Another problem is misunderstanding or misinterpreting the kind of sexual statement you want to make. What is a sexual statement? Even asking the question is confusing. Surely there is a wide gap between Madonna and Joan Collins, Michelle Pfeiffer and Iman, or Glenn Close (particularly in *Fatal Attraction*) and Kathleen Turner (particularly in *Body Heat*.) All these women represent a totally different sexual statement and each one wears a strikingly different makeup application. That's not to say that any one of them has more sex appeal than another; we are only talking about the external image makeup (and clothing for that matter) can project.

Developing sex appeal is not the point of this book, but I would be remiss not to acknowledge that looking more alluring to attract the opposite sex is part of why some women wear makeup. Creating that image requires balance and realistic expectations. As I have said all along, more makeup is not necessarily more sexy; balance is definitely the way to approach how you dress your face regardless of the intent. The bottom line is that what we want is sometimes confused or hindered by our makeup and sometimes accentuated. There are times where I feel more sexy with a full makeup on, but there are also times where that much makeup feels heavy and like a mask.

For the last few words I have with you, I'm not going to recommend ways to keep your makeup on throughout the night and how to touch up after an active night together so he doesn't see you without your makeup on. Rather, I'm going to remind you that how sexy or powerful someone wants to be is only possible when they choose to be sexy or powerful. Clothing and makeup can portray certain images, but makeup is only a tool, an accessory, that can creatively be used to your best advantage or disadvantage. It's up to you.

Index